MW00463762

Copyright © 2021 by Emanuel Kirby -All rights reserved.

No part of this publication may be reproduced, distributed, or transmitted in any form or by any means, including photocopying, recording, or other electronic or mechanical methods, without the prior written permission of the publisher, except in the case of brief quotations embodied in reviews and certain other non-commercial uses permitted by copyright law.

This Book is provided with the sole purpose of providing relevant information on a specific topic for which every reasonable effort has been made to ensure that it is both accurate and reasonable. Nevertheless, by purchasing this Book you consent to the fact that the author, as well as the publisher, are in no way experts on the topics contained herein, regardless of any claims as such that may be made within. It is recommended that you always consult a professional prior to undertaking any of the advice or techniques discussed within.This is a legally binding declaration that is considered both valid and fair by both the Committee of Publishers Association and the American Bar Association and should be considered as legally binding within the United States.

CONTENTS

VEGETARIAN & VEGAN RECIPES

Braised Swiss Chard With Lime

Servings: 2
Cooking Time: 25 Minutes
Ingredients:
- 2 pounds Swiss chard
- 4 tbsp of extra virgin olive oil
- 2 garlic cloves, crushed
- 1 whole lime, juiced
- 2 tsps sea salt

Directions:
1. Thoroughly rinse Swiss chard and drain in a colander. Using a sharp paring knife roughly chop and transfer to a large bowl. Stir in 4 tablespoons of olive oil, crushed garlic, lime juice, and sea salt. Transfer to a large vacuum-sealable bag and seal. Cook en sous vide for 10 minutes at 180 F.

White Beans

Servings: 8
Cooking Time: 3-4 Hours
Ingredients:
- 1 cup dried and soaked navy beans
- 1 cup water
- ½ cup extra-virgin olive oil
- 1 peeled carrot, cut up into 1-inch dices
- 1 stalk celery, cut up into 1-inch dices
- 1 quartered shallot
- 4 cloves crushed garlic
- 2 sprigs fresh rosemary
- 2 pieces' bay leaves
- Kosher salt, to taste
- Freshly ground black pepper, to taste

Directions:
1. Prepare your Sous-vide water bath using your immersion circulator and raise the temperature to 190-degrees Fahrenheit.
2. Carefully drain and rinse your beans and add them alongside the rest of the ingredients to a heavy-duty zip bag.
3. Seal using the immersion method and submerge it underwater. Cook for about 3 hours.
4. Once cooked, taste the beans.

5. If they are firm, then cook for another 1 hour and pour them in a serving bowl.
6. Serve!
Nutrition Info: Per serving:Calories: 210 ;Carbohydrates: 36g ;Protein: 14g ;Fat: 2g ;Sugar: 2g ;Sodium: 224mg

Paprika Grits

Servings: 4
Cooking Time: 3 Hours 10 Minutes
Ingredients:
- 10 ounces grits
- 4 tbsp butter
- 1 ½ tsp paprika
- 10 ounces water
- ½ tsp garlic salt

Directions:
1. Prepare a water bath and place the Sous Vide in it. Set to 180 F.
2. Place all the ingredients in a vacumm-sealable bag. Stir with spoon to combine well. Release air by the water displacement method, seal and submerge the bag in water bath.Set the timer for 3 hours. Once the timer has stopped, remove the bag. Divide between 4 serving bowls.

Grape Vegetable Mix

Servings: 9
Cooking Time: 105 Minutes
Ingredients:
- 8 sweet potatoes, sliced
- 2 red onions, sliced
- 4 ounces tomato, pureed
- 1 tsp minced garlic
- Salt and black pepper to taste
- 1 tsp grape juice

Directions:
1. Prepare a water bath and place Sous Vide in it. Set to 183 F. Place all the ingredients with ¼ cup water in a vacumm-sealable bag.Release air by the water displacement method, seal and submerge the

bag in water bath. Set the timer for 90 minutes. Once the timer has stopped, remove the bag. Serve warm.

Herby Balsamic Mushrooms With Garlic

Servings: 4
Cooking Time: 1 Hour 15 Minutes
Ingredients:

- 1 pound Portobello mushrooms, sliced
- 1 tbsp olive oil
- 1 tbsp apple balsamic vinegar
- 1 minced garlic clove
- Salt to taste
- 1 tsp black pepper
- 1 tsp minced fresh thyme

Directions:
1. Prepare a water bath and place the Sous Vide in it. Set to 138 F.
2. Combine all the ingredients and place them in a vacuum-sealable bag. Release air by the water displacement method, seal and submerge the bag in the water bath. Cook for 60 minutes. Once the timer has stopped, remove the bag and transfer to a serving bowl.

Shallot Cabbage With Raisins

Servings: 4
Cooking Time: 2 Hours 15 Minutes
Ingredients:

- 1 ½ pounds red cabbage, sliced
- ¼ cup raisins
- 2 sliced shallots
- 3 sliced garlic cloves
- 1 tbsp apple balsamic vinegar
- 1 tbsp butter

Directions:
1. Prepare a water bath and place Sous Vide in it. Set to 186 F. Place the cabbage in a vacuum-sealable bag. Add the reamaining ingredients. Release air by the water displacement method, seal and submerge the bag in the water bath. Cook for 2 hours. Once the timer has stopped, remove the bags and transfer into serving bowls. Season with salt and vinegar. Top with the cooking juices.

Celery & Leek Potato Soup

Servings: 8
Cooking Time: 2 Hours 15 Minutes
Ingredients:

- 8 tbsp butter
- 4 red potatoes, sliced
- 1 yellow onion, cut into ¼-inch pieces
- 1 celery stalk, cut into ½-inch pieces
- 4 cups ½-inch diced leeks, white parts only
- 1 cup vegetable stock
- 1 carrot, chopped
- 4 garlic cloves, minced
- 2 bay leaves
- Salt and black pepper to taste
- 2 cups heavy cream
- ¼ cup chopped fresh chives

Directions:
1. Prepare a water bath and place the Sous Vide in it. Set to 186 F.
2. Place the potatoes, carrots, onion, celery, leeks, vegetable stock, butter, garlic, and bay leaves in a vacuum-sealable bag. Release air by the water displacement method, seal and submerge the bag in the water bath. Cook for 2 hours.
3. Once the timer has stopped, remove the bag and transfer into a blender. Discard the bay leaves. Mix the contents and season with salt and pepper. Pour the cream slowly and blend 2-3 minutes until smooth. Drain the contents and garnish with chives to serve.

Spicy Giardiniera

Servings: 8
Cooking Time: 60 Minutes
Ingredients:

- 2 cups white wine vinegar
- 1 cup water
- ½ cup beet sugar
- 3 tablespoons kosher salt
- 1 tablespoon whole black peppercorns
- 1 cup cauliflower, cut up into ½-inch pieces
- 1 stemmed and seeded bell pepper, cut up into ½-inch pieces
- 1 cup carrots, cut up into ½-inch pieces
- ½ thinly sliced white onion

- 2 seeded and stemmed Serrano peppers, cut up into ½-inch pieces

Directions:

1. Prepare the Sous-vide water bath using your immersion circulator and raise the temperature to 180-degrees Fahrenheit.
2. Take a large bowl and mix in vinegar, sugar, salt, water, and peppercorns.
3. Transfer the mixture to a large resealable zipper bag and add the cauliflower, onion, serrano peppers, vinegar mixture, bell pepper, and carrots.
4. Seal it up using the immersion method and submerge underwater, cook for about 1 hour.
5. Once cooked, take it out from the bag and serve

Nutrition Info: Per serving:Calories: 245 ;Carbohydrates: 42g ;Protein: 4g ;Fat: 7g ;Sugar: 30g ;Sodium: 640mg

Vegetarian Parmesan Risotto

Servings: 5
Cooking Time: 65 Minutes
Ingredients:
- 2 cups Arborio rice
- ½ cup plain white rice
- 1 cup veggie stock
- 1 cup water
- 6-8 ounces Parmesan cheese, grated
- 1 onion, chopped
- 1 tbsp butter
- Salt and black pepper to taste

Directions:

1. Prepare a water bath and place Sous Vide in it. Set to 185 F. Melt the butter in a saucepan over medium heat. Add onions, rice and spices and cook for a few minutes. Transfer to a vacuum-sealable bag. Release air by the water displacement method, seal and submerge the bag in water bath. Set the timer for 50 minutes. Once the timer has stopped, remove the bag ans stir in the Parmesan cheese.

Honey Drizzled Carrots

Servings: 4
Cooking Time: 75 Minutes
Ingredients:

- 1-pound baby carrots
- 4 tablespoons vegan butter
- 1 tablespoon agave nectar
- 3 tablespoons honey
- ¼ teaspoon kosher salt
- ¼ teaspoon ground cardamom

Directions:

1. Prepare the Sous-vide water bath using your immersion circulator and increase the temperature to 185 degrees Fahrenheit
2. Add the carrots, honey, whole butter, kosher salt, and cardamom to a resealable bag
3. Seal using the immersion method. Cook for 75 minutes and once done, remove it from the water bath.
4. Strain the glaze by passing through a fine mesh.
5. Set it aside.
6. Take the carrots out from the bag and pour any excess glaze over them. Serve with a little bit of seasonings.

Nutrition Info: Per serving:Calories: 174 ;Carbohydrates: 42g ;Protein: 2g ;Fat: 1g ;Sugar: 31g ;Sodium: 180mg

Beet Spinach Salad

Servings: 3
Cooking Time: 2 Hours 25 Minutes
Ingredients:
- 1 ¼ cup beets, trimmed and cut into bite-sized pieces
- 1 cup fresh spinach, chopped
- 2 tbsp olive oil
- 1 tbsp lemon juice, freshly juiced
- 1 tsp balsamic vinegar
- 2 garlic cloves, crushed
- 1 tbsp butter
- Salt and black pepper to taste

Directions:

1. Rinse well and clean beets. Chop into bite-sized pieces and place in a vacuum-sealable bag along with butter and crushed garlic. Cook in Sous Vide for 2 hours at 185 F. Set aside to cool.
2. Boil a large pot of water and place spinach in it. Cook for one minute, and then remove from the heat. Drain well. Transfer to a vacuum-sealable bag and

cook in Sous Vide for 10 minutes at 180 F. Remove from the water bath and cool completely. Place in a large bowl and add cooked beets. Season with salt, pepper, vinegar, olive oil, and lemon juice. Serve immediately.

Chili Garbanzo Bean Stew

Servings: 4
Cooking Time: 3 Hours 10 Minutes
Ingredients:
- 1 cup garbanzo beans, soaked overnight
- 3 cups water
- 1 tbsp olive oil
- Salt to taste
- ½ tsp ground cumin
- ½ tsp ground coriander
- ¼ tsp ground cinnamon
- 1/8 tsp ground cloves
- 1/8 tsp cayenne pepper
- Chopped fresh cilantro
- Harissa sauce, to taste

Directions:
1. Prepare a water bath and place the Sous Vide in it. Set to 192 F.
2. Place beans in a vacuum-sealable bag with cumin, salt, olive oil, cloves, cinnamon, cilantro, and cayenne. Release air by water displacement method, seal and submerge in the water bath. Cook for 3 hours. Once done, remove the bag and drain the beans. Discard the cooking juices. Season with salt. Combine the olive oil and harissa sauce and pour over the beans. Garnish with cilantro.

Long Green Beans In Tomato Sauce

Servings: 4
Cooking Time: 3 Hours
Ingredients:
- 1 pound, trimmed green beans
- 1 can, whole crushed tomatoes
- 1 thinly sliced onion
- 3 peeled and thinly sliced garlic clove
- Kosher salt as needed
- Extra virgin olive oil

Directions:

1. Prepare your Sous Vide water bath by dipping your immersion cooker and raising the temperature to 183ºF
2. Take a heavy-duty zip bag and add tomatoes, green bean, garlic, and onion
3. Submerge underwater and cook for 3 hours
4. Remove the bag and transfer content to a large sized bowl
5. Season with salt and drizzle a bit of olive oil
6. Serve and enjoy!
Nutrition Info: Per serving:Calories 54, Carbohydrates 5 g, Fats 2 g, Protein 4 g

Honey Apple & Arugula Salad

Servings: 4
Cooking Time: 3 Hours 50 Minutes
Ingredients:
- 2 tbsp honey
- 2 apples, cored, halved and sliced
- ½ cup walnuts, toasted and chopped
- ½ cup shaved Grana Padano cheese
- 4 cups arugula
- Sea salt to taste
- Dressing
- ¼ cup olive oil
- 1 tbsp white wine vinegar
- 1 tsp Dijon mustard
- 1 garlic clove, minced
- Salt to taste

Directions:
1. Prepare a water bath and place the Sous Vide in it. Set to 158 F. Place the honey in a glass bowl and heat for 30 seconds, add the apples and mix well. Place it in a vacuum-sealable bag. Release air by the water displacement method, seal and submerge the bag in the water bath. Cook for 30 minutes.
2. Once the timer has stopped, remove the bag and transfer into an ice-water bath for 5 minutes. Refrigerate for 3 hours. Combine all the dressing ingredients in a jar and shake well. Allow cooling in the fridge for a moment.
3. In a bowl, mix the arugula, walnuts, and Grana Padano cheese. Add the peach slices. Top with the dressing. Season with salt and pepper and serve.

Fall Squash Cream Soup

Servings: 6
Cooking Time: 2 Hours 20 Minutes
Ingredients:
- ¾ cup heavy cream
- 1 winter squash, chopped
- 1 large pear
- ½ yellow onion, diced
- 3 fresh thyme sprigs
- 1 garlic clove, chopped
- 1 tsp ground cumin
- Salt and black pepper to taste
- 4 tbsp crème fraîche

Directions:
1. Prepare a water bath and place the Sous Vide in it. Set to 186 F.
2. Combine the squash, pear, onion, thyme, garlic, cumin, and salt. Place in a vacuum-sealable bag. Release air by the water displacement method, seal and submerge in water bath. Cook for 2 hours.
3. Once the timer has stopped, remove the bag and transfer all the contents into a blender. Puree until smooth. Add in cream and stir well. Season with salt and pepper. Transfer the mix into serving bowls and top with some créme fraiche. Garnish with pear chunks.

Oregano White Beans

Servings: 8
Cooking Time: 5 Hours 15 Minutes
Ingredients:
- 12 ounces white beans
- 1 cup tomato paste
- 8 ounces veggie stock
- 1 tbsp sugar
- 3 tbsp butter
- 1 cup chopped onions
- 1 bell pepper, chopped
- 1 tbsp oregano
- 2 tsp paprika

Directions:
1. Prepare a water bath and place the Sous Vide in it. Set to 185 F.
2. Combine all the ingredients in a vacumm-sealable bag. Stir to combine. Release air by the

water displacement method, seal and submerge the bag in water bath.Set the timer for 5 hours. Once the timer has stopped, remove the bag. Serve warm.

Allspice Miso Corn With Sesame & Honey

Servings: 4
Cooking Time: 45 Minutes
Ingredients:
- 4 ears of corn
- 6 tbsp butter
- 3 tbsp red miso paste
- 1 tsp honey
- 1 tsp allspice
- 1 tbsp canola oil
- 1 scallion, thinly sliced
- 1 tsp toasted sesame seeds

Directions:
1. Prepare a water bath and place the Sous Vide in it. Set to 183 F. Clean the corn and cut the ears. Cover each corn with 2 tbsp of butter. Place in a vacuum-sealable bag. Release air by the water displacement method, seal and submerge the bag in the water bath. Cook for 30 minutes.
2. Meanwhile, combine 4 tbsp of butter, 2 tbsp of miso paste, honey, canola oil, and allspice in a bowl. Stir well. Set aside. Once the timer has stopped, remove the bag and sear the corn. Spread the miso mixture on top. Garnish with sesame oil and scallions.

Flavorful Vegan Stew With Cannellini Beans

Servings: 8
Cooking Time: 3 Hours 15 Minutes
Ingredients:
- 1 cup cannellini beans, soaked overnight
- 1 cup water
- ½ cup olive oil
- 1 peeled carrot, chopped
- 1 stalk celery, chopped
- 1 quartered shallot
- 4 cloves crushed garlic
- 2 sprigs fresh rosemary
- 2 bay leaves

- Salt and black pepper to taste

Directions:

1. Prepare a water bath and place the Sous Vide in it. Set to 192 F.

2. Strain and wash the beans and place with the remaining ingredients in a vacuum-sealable bag. Release air by the water displacement method, seal and submerge the bag in the water bath. Cook for 3 hours.

3. Once the timer has stopped, remove the bag and dash the consistency. If you want more soften cook for another 1 hour. When done, transfer into a bowl.

Broiled Onions With Sunflower Pesto

Servings: 4

Cooking Time: 2 Hours 25 Minutes

Ingredients:

- 1 bunch large spring onions, trimmed and halved
- ½ cup plus 2 tbsp olive oil
- Salt and black pepper to taste
- 2 tbsp sunflower seeds
- 2 cloves garlic, peeled
- 3 cups loosely packed fresh basil leaves
- 3 tbsp grated Grana Padano cheese
- 1 tbsp freshly squeezed lemon juice

Directions:

1. Prepare a water bath and place the Sous Vide in it. Set to 183 F.

2. Place the onions in a vacuum-sealable bag. Season with salt, pepper and 2 tbsp of olive oil. Release air by the water displacement method, seal and submerge the bag in the water bath. Cook for 2 hours.

3. Meanwhile, for the pesto sauce, combine in a processor food the sunflower seeds, garlic, and basil, and blend until finely chopped. Carefully add the remaining oil. Add in lemon juice and stop. Season with salt and pepper. Set aside.

4. Once the timer has stopped, remove the bag and transfer the onions to a skillet and cook for 10 minutes. Serve and top with the pesto sauce.

Creamy Gnocchi With Peas

Servings: 2

Cooking Time: 1 Hour 50 Minutes

Ingredients:

- 1 pack gnocchi
- 1 tbsp butter
- ½ thinly sliced sweet onion
- Salt and black pepper to taste
- ½ cup frozen peas
- ¼ cup heavy cream
- ½ cup grated Pecorino Romano cheese

Directions:

1. Prepare a water bath and place the Sous Vide in it. Set to 183 F. Place the gnocchi in a vacuum-sealable bag. Release air by the water displacement method, seal and submerge the bag in the water bath. Cook for 1 hour and 30 minutes.

2. Once the timer has stopped, remove the bag and set aside. Heat a skillet over medium heat with butter and sauté the onion for 3 minutes. Add the frozen peas and cream and cook. Combine the gnocchi with the cream sauce, season with pepper and salt and serve in a plate.

Sous Vide Balsamic Onions

Servings: 2

Cooking Time: 2 Hours

Ingredients:

- 2 medium white onions, sliced julienne
- 1 tbsp, balsamic vinegar
- 2 tbsp, brown sugar
- 2 tbsp, olive oil
- Salt/Pepper to taste

Directions:

1. Prepare your Sous Vide water bath by attaching the immersion circulator and setting the temperature to 185ºF.

2. Mix the onions with the rest of the ingredients in a sealable plastic bag and seal using a vacuum sealer or the water displacement method.

3. Submerge into the bath water and allow cooking for 2 hours.

4. Remove, transfer into a mason jar, cool and keep in the fridge for up to 12 hours before serving.

Nutrition Info: Per serving:Calories 186.7, Carbohydrates 15.5 g, Fats 13.5 g, Protein 0.8 g

Mixed Beans In Tomato Sauce

Servings: 4
Cooking Time: 3 Hours 10 Minutes
Ingredients:
- 1 pound trimmed green beans
- 1 pound trimmed snow beans
- 1 (14-oz) can whole crushed tomatoes
- 1 thinly sliced onion
- 3 sliced garlic cloves
- 3 tbsp olive oil

Directions:
1. Prepare a water bath and place Sous Vide in it. Set to 183 F. Place the tomatoes, snow and green beans, garlic, and onion in a vacuum-sealable bag. Release air by water displacement method, seal and submerge in the water bath. Cook for 3 hours. Once done, transfer into a bowl. Sprinkle with olive oil.

Sweet Red Beet Dish

Servings: 4
Cooking Time: 1 Hour 45 Minutes
Ingredients:
- 1 pound red beets, peeled and quartered
- 2 tbsp butter
- 2 peeled oranges, chopped
- 1 tbsp honey
- 3 tbsp balsamic vinegar
- 4 tbsp olive oil
- Salt and black pepper to taste
- 6 oz baby romaine leaves
- ½ cup pistachios, chopped
- ½ cup Pecorino Romano cheese

Directions:
1. Prepare a water bath and place the Sous Vide in it. Set to 182 F.
2. Place the red beets in a vacuum-sealable bag. Add the butter Release air by the water displacement method, seal and submerge the bag in the water bath. Cook for 90 minutes.
3. Once the timer has stopped, remove the bag and discard the cooking juices. Combine the honey, oil and vinegar. Season with salt and pepper. Throw the romaine leaves, orange, beets, and vinaigrette. Garnish with pistachio and Pecorino Romano cheese.

Spicy Black Beans

Servings: 6
Cooking Time: 6 Hours 15 Minutes
Ingredients:
- 1 cup dry black beans
- 3 cups water
- 1/3 cup lemon juice
- 2 tbsp lemon zest
- Salt to taste
- 1 tsp cumin
- ½ tsp chipotle chili powder

Directions:
1. Prepare a water bath and place Sous Vide in it. Set to 193 F. Place all the ingredients in a vacuum-sealable bag. Release air by the water displacement method, seal and submerge the bag in the water bath. Cook for 6 hours. Once the timer has stopped, remove the bag and transfer into a hot saucepan over medium heat and cook until reduced. Remove from the heat and serve.

Sous Vide Turmeric And Cumin Tofu

Servings: 4
Cooking Time: 2 Hours
Ingredients:
- 1 pack, firm tofu, drained and cut to ½ inch thick pieces
- 3 cloves, garlic, minced
- 1 tbsp, turmeric
- 1 tsp, cumin
- 2 tbsp, lime
- 3 tablespoons olive oil
- Kosher salt/Pepper

Directions:
1. Prepare your Sous Vide water bath by attaching the immersion circulator and setting the temperature to 180ºF.
2. Arrange the tofu pieces on a flat surface (you can use a baking tray) and place on the fridge for 15 minutes.

3. In a small bowl, combine all the rest of the ingredients to make a marinade.

4. Take the tofu pieces out of the fridge and dip into the marinade, making sure all pieces are well coated.

5. Transfer the marinated tofu on a sealable pouch (lying flat) and seal using a vacuum sealer or the water displacement method.

6. Submerge into the water bath and let cook for 2 hours.

7. Take out of the pouch carefully and serve as it is or with lettuce or Roca leaves as a garnish.

Nutrition Info: Per serving:Calories 220, Carbohydrates 5.4 g, Fats 16.9 g, Protein 11.7 g

Curry Ginger & Nectarine Chutney

Servings: 3
Cooking Time: 60 Minutes
Ingredients:
- ½ cup granulated sugar
- ½ cup water
- ¼ cup white wine vinegar
- 1 garlic clove, minced
- ¼ cup white onion, finely chopped
- Juice of 1 lime
- 2 tsp grated fresh ginger
- 2 tsp curry powder
- A pinch of red pepper flakes
- Salt and black pepper to taste
- Pepper flakes to taste
- 4 large pieces nectarine, sliced into wedges
- ¼ cup chopped up fresh basil

Directions:
1. Prepare a water bath and place the Sous Vide in it. Set to 168 F.

2. Heat a saucepan over medium heat and combine the water, sugar, white wine vinegar, and garlic. Moving until the sugar soften. Add lime juice, onion, curry powder, ginger, and red pepper flakes. Season with salt and black pepper. Stir well. Place the mixture in a vacuum-sealable bag. Release air by the water displacement method, seal and submerge the bag in the water bath. Cook for 40 minutes.

3. Once the timer has stopped, remove the bag and place in ice bath. Transfer the food on a serving plate. Garnish with basil.

Delicious Cardamom And Apricots

Servings: 4
Cooking Time: 1 Hour
Ingredients:
- 1 pint, mall and halved apricots
- 1 tablespoon, unsalted butter
- 1 teaspoon, cardamom seeds freshly ground
- ½ a teaspoon, ground ginger
- Just a pinch, smoked sea salt
- Chopped up fresh basil

Directions:
1. Prepare your Sous Vide water bath by increasing the temperature to a 180ºF using an immersion cooker

2. Take a large sized heavy-duty plastic bag and add butter, apricots, ginger, cardamom, salt and mix the whole mixture well

3. Seal up the bag using water displacement method and submerge it underwater

4. Let it cook for 1 hour and remove the bag once done

5. Take serving bowls and add the apricots to the bowl

6. Garnish with a bit of basil and serve!

Nutrition Info: Per serving:Calories 28, Carbohydrates 6 g, Fats 0 g, Protein 1 g

Tomato & Agave Tofu

Servings: 6
Cooking Time: 1 Hour 45 Minutes
Ingredients:
- 1 cup vegetable broth
- 2 tbsp tomato paste
- 1 tbsp turmeric powder
- 1 tbsp rice wine vinegar
- 1 tbsp agave nectar
- 2 tsp sriracha sauce
- 3 cloves minced garlic
- 1 tsp soy sauce
- 24 oz silken tofu, cubed

Directions:

1. Prepare a water bath and place the Sous Vide in it. Set to 186 F. Combine all the ingredients in a bowl, except the tofu.
2. Place the tofu in a vacuum-sealable bag. Add the mixture. Release air by the water displacement method, seal and submerge the bag in the water bath. Cook for 1 hour and 30 minutes. Once the timer has stopped, remove the bag. Serve.

Truffle Sunchokes

Servings: 4
Cooking Time: 90 Minutes
Ingredients:
- 8 ounces peeled Sunchokes, sliced into ¼ inch thick pieces
- 3 tablespoons unsalted vegan butter
- 2 tablespoons agave nectar
- 1 teaspoon truffle oil
- Kosher salt, and black pepper, to taste

Directions:
1. Prepare the Sous Vide water bath using your immersion circulator and raise the temperature to 180-degrees Fahrenheit.
2. Take a heavy-duty resealable zip bag and add the butter, nectar, sunchokes, truffle oil and mix them well.
3. Sprinkle some salt and pepper, and then seal using the immersion method.
4. Submerge it underwater and cook for 1 ½ hour.
5. Once cooked, transfer the contents to a skillet.
6. Put the skillet over medium-high heat and cook for 5 minutes more until the liquid has evaporated.
7. Season with pepper and salt to adjust the flavor if needed
8. Serve!

Nutrition Info: Per serving:Calories: 255 ;Carbohydrates: 40g ;Protein: 5g ;Fat: 10g ;Sugar: 22g ;Sodium: 360mg

Simple Broccoli Rabe

Servings: 2
Cooking Time: 20 Minutes
Ingredients:
- ½ pound broccoli rabe
- 1 tsp garlic powder
- 1 tbsp vegan butter

- ½ tsp sea salt
- ¼ tsp black pepper

Directions:
1. Prepare a water bath and place the Sous Vide in it. Set to 192 F.
2. Place the broccoli rabe, garlic powder, sea salt, and black pepper in a vacuum-sealable bag. Release air by the water displacement method, seal and submerge the bag in the water bath. Cook for 4 minutes. Once the timer has stopped, remove the broccoli to a serving plate.

Vegetable Caponata

Servings: 4
Cooking Time: 2 Hours 15 Minutes
Ingredients:
- 4 canned plum tomatoes, crushed
- 2 bell peppers, sliced
- 2 zucchinis, sliced
- ½ onion, sliced
- 2 eggplants, sliced
- 6 garlic cloves, minced
- 2 tbsp olive oil
- 6 basil leaves
- Salt and black pepper to taste

Directions:
1. Prepare a water bath and place the Sous Vide in it. Set to 185 F. Combine all of the ingredients in a vacumm-sealable bag. Release air by the water displacement method, seal and submerge the bag in water bath.Set the timer for 2 hours. Once the timer has stopped, transfer to a serving platter.

Ginger Tamari Brussels Sprouts With Sesame

Servings: 6
Cooking Time: 43 Minutes
Ingredients:
- 1½ pounds Brussels sprouts, halved
- 2 garlic cloves, minced
- 2 tbsp vegetable oil
- 1 tbsp tamari sauce
- 1 tsp grated ginger
- ¼ tsp red pepper flakes
- ¼ tsp toasted sesame oil

- 1 tbsp sesame seeds

Directions:

1. Prepare a water bath and place Sous Vide in it. Set to 186 F. Heat a pot over medium heat and combine the garlic, vegetable oil, tamari sauce, ginger, and red pepper flakes. Cook for 4-5 minutes. Set aside.

2. Place the brussels sprouts in a vacuum-sealable bag and pour in tamari mixture. Release air by the water displacement method, seal and submerge the bag in the water bath. Cook for 30 minutes.

3. Once the timer has stopped, remove the bag and pat dry with kitchen towel. Reserve the cooking juices. Transfer the sprouts to a bowl and combine with the sesame oil. Plate the sprouts and sprinkle with cooking juices. Garnish with sesame seeds.

Cabbage Wedges

Servings: 2

Cooking Time: 4 Hours

Ingredients:

- 1 medium-sized savoy cabbage cut up into wedges
- 2 tablespoons, unsalted butter
- ½ teaspoon, kosher salt

Directions:

1. Prepare your Sous Vide water bath by dipping your immersion cooker and raising the temperature to 183ºF

2. Take a large sized zip bag and add 1 tablespoon of butter, salt, and cabbages

3. Mix well and seal using immersion method

4. Cook for 4 hours and remove the cabbage, pat dry using kitchen towel

5. Take a tablespoon of butter and add to a medium-sized skillet over medium heat

6. Allow the butter to melt and add cabbages

7. Sear for 5-7 minutes until golden

8. Serve and enjoy!

Nutrition Info: Per serving:Calories 42, Carbohydrates 4 g, Fats 2 g, Protein 2 g

Provolone Cheese Grits

Servings: 4

Cooking Time: 3 Hours 20 Minutes

Ingredients:

- 1 cup grits
- 1 cup cream
- 3 cups vegetable stock
- 2 tbsp butter
- 4 oz grated Provolone cheese
- 1 tbsp paprika
- Extra cheese for garnish
- Salt and black pepper to taste

Directions:

1. Prepare a water bath and place the Sous Vide in it. Set to 182 F. Combine the grits, cream and vegetable stock. Chop the butter and add to the mixture. Place the mix in a vacuum-sealable bag. Release air by the water displacement method, seal and submerge the bag in the water bath. Cook for 3 hours.

2. Once the timer has stopped, remove the bag and transfer into a bowl. Stir the mixture with the cheese and season with salt and pepper. Garnish with extra cheese and paprika, if preferred.

Easy Vegetable Alfredo Dressing

Servings: 6

Cooking Time: 1 Hour 45 Minutes

Ingredients:

- 4 cups chopped cauliflower
- 2 cups water
- 2/3 cup hazelnuts
- 2 cloves garlic
- ½ tsp dried oregano
- ½ tsp dried basil
- ½ tsp dried rosemary
- 4 tbsp nutritional yeast
- Salt and black pepper to taste

Directions:

1. Prepare a water bath and place the Sous Vide in it. Set to 172 F.

2. Place the hazelnuts, cauliflower, oregano, water, garlic, rosemary, and basil in a vacuum-sealable bag. Release air by the water displacement method, seal and submerge the bag in the water bath. Cook for 90 minutes.

3. Once the timer has stopped, remove the contents and transfer into a blender and blend until pureed. Serve with pasta.

Cream Of Tomatoes With Cheese Sandwich

Servings: 8
Cooking Time: 55 Minutes
Ingredients:

- ½ cup cream cheese
- 2 pounds tomatoes, cut into wedges
- Salt and black pepper to taste
- 2 tbsp olive oil
- 2 garlic cloves, minced
- ½ tsp chopped fresh sage
- ⅛ tsp red pepper flakes
- ½ tsp white wine vinegar
- 2 tbsp butter
- 4 slices bread
- 2 slices halloumi cheese

Directions:

1. Prepare a water bath and place the Sous Vide in it. Set to 186 F. Put the tomatoes in a colander over a bowl and season with salt. Stir well. Allow to chill for 30 minutes. Discard the juices. Combine the olive oil, garlic, sage, black pepper, salt, and pepper flakes.
2. Place in a vacuum-sealable bag. Release air by the water displacement method, seal and submerge the bag in the water bath. Cook for 40 minutes.
3. Once the timer has stopped, remove the bag and transfer into a blender. Add in vinegar and cream cheese. Mix until smooth. Transfer to a plate and season with salt and pepper if needed.
4. To make the cheese bars: heat a skillet over medium heat. Grease the bread slices with butter and put into the skillet. Lay cheese slices over the bread and place over another buttery bread. Toast for 1-2 minutes. Repeat with the remaining bread. Cut into cubes. Serve over the warm soup.

Maple Beet Salad With Cashews & Queso Fresco

Servings: 8
Cooking Time: 1 Hour 35 Minutes
Ingredients:

- 6 large beets, peeled and cut into chunks
- Salt and black pepper to taste
- 3 tbsp maple syrup
- 2 tbsp butter
- Zest of 1 large orange
- 1 tbsp olive oil
- ½ tsp cayenne pepper
- 1½ cups cashews
- 6 cup arugula
- 3 tangerines, peeled and segmented
- 1 cup queso fresco, crumbled

Directions:

1. Prepare a water bath and place the Sous Vide in it. Set to 186 F.
2. Place the beet chunks in a vacuum-sealable bag. Season with salt and pepper. Add 2 tbsp of maple syrup, butter, and orange zest. Release air by the water displacement method, seal and submerge the bag in the water bath. Cook for 1 hour and 15 minutes.
3. Preheat the oven to 350 F.
4. Mix the remaining maple syrup, olive oil, salt, and cayenne. Add in cashews and stir well. Transfer the cashew mixture into a baking tray, previously lined with wax pepper and bake for 10 minutes. Set aside and allow to cool.
5. Once the timer has stopped, remove the beets and discard the cooking juices. Put the arugula on a serving plate, beets and tangerine wedges all over. Scatter with queso fresco and cashew mix to serve.

Tasty Spicy Tomatoes

Servings: 4
Cooking Time: 60 Minutes
Ingredients:

- 4 pieces cored and diced tomatoes
- 2 tbsp olive oil
- 3 minced garlic cloves
- 1 tsp dried oregano
- 1 tsp rosemary
- 1 tsp fine sea salt

Directions:

1. Prepare a water bath and place Sous Vide in it. Set to 146 F. Place all the ingredients in a vacuum-sealable bag. Release air by the water displacement method, seal and submerge in the bath. Cook for 45 minutes. Once the timer has stopped, remove the tomatoes and transfer to a plate. Serve with toast French bread slices.

Hearty White Beans

Servings: 8
Cooking Time: 3 Hours
Ingredients:
- 1 cup, dried and soaked navy beans
- 1 cup, water
- ½ a cup, extra virgin olive oil
- 1 peeled carrot cut up into 1-inch dices
- 1 stalk, celery cut up into 1-inch dices
- 1 quartered shallot
- 4 cloves, crushed garlic
- 2 sprigs, fresh rosemary
- 2 pieces, bay leaves
- Kosher salt
- Freshly ground black pepper

Directions:
1. Prepare your Sous Vide water bath by dipping your immersion cooker and raising the temperature to 190ºF
2. Carefully drain and rinse your beans and add them to a heavy-duty zipper bag
3. Seal it up using immersion method and submerge it underwater
4. Let it cook for about 3 hours
5. Once done, taste the beans
6. If they are firm, then cook for another 1 hour, or cook for another hour and serve them on a bowl
7. Serve!

Nutrition Info: Per serving:Calories 119, Carbohydrates 9 g, Fats 3 g, Protein 14 g

Cilantro Turmeric Quinoa

Servings: 6
Cooking Time: 105 Minutes
Ingredients:
- 3 cups quinoa
- 2 cups heavy cream
- ½ cup water
- 3 tbsp cilantro leaves
- 2 tsp turmeric powder
- 1 tbsp butter
- ½ tbsp salt

Directions:
1. Prepare a water bath and place the Sous Vide in it. Set to 180 F.
2. Place all the ingredients in a vacumm-sealable bag. Stir to combine well. Release air by the water

displacement method, seal and submerge the bag in water bath. Set the timer for 90 minutes. Once the timer has stopped, remove the bag. Serve warm.

Green Pea Cream With Nutmeg

Servings: 8
Cooking Time: 1 Hour 10 Minutes
Ingredients:
- 1 pound fresh green peas
- 1 cup whipping cream
- ¼ cup butter
- 1 tbsp cornstarch
- ¼ tsp ground nutmeg
- 4 cloves
- 2 bay leaves
- Black pepper to taste

Directions:
1. Prepare a water bath and place the Sous Vide in it. Set to 184 F. Combine the cornstarch, nutmeg and cream into a bowl. Whisk until the cornstarch soften.
2. Place the mixture in a vacuum-sealable bag. Release air by the water displacement method, seal and submerge the bag in the water bath. Cook for 1 hour. Once the timer has stopped, extract the bag and remove the bay leaf. Serve.

Root Veggie Mash

Servings: 4
Cooking Time: 3 Hours 15 Minutes
Ingredients:
- 2 parsnips, peeled and chopped
- 1 turnip, peeled and chopped
- 1 large sweet potatoes, peeled and chopped
- 1 tbsp butter
- Salt and black pepper to taste
- Pinch of nutmeg
- ¼ tsp thyme

Directions:
1. Prepare a water bath and place Sous Vide in it. Set to 185 F. Place the veggies in a vacumm-sealable bag. Release air by the water displacement method, seal and submerge in water bath.Cook for 3 hours. Once done, remove the bag and mash the veggies with a potato masher. Stir in the remaining ingredients.

Eggplant Lasagna

Servings: 3
Cooking Time: 3 Hours
Ingredients:

- 1 lb eggplants, peeled and thinly sliced
- 1 tsp salt
- 1 cup tomato sauce, divided into 3
- 2 oz fresh mozzarella, thinly sliced
- 1 oz Parmesan cheese, grated
- 2 oz Italian blend cheese, grated
- 3 tbsp fresh basil, chopped
- Topping:
- ½ tbsp macadamia nuts, toasted and chopped
- 1 oz Parmesan cheese, grated
- 1 oz italian blend cheese, grated

Directions:

1. Make a water bath, place Sous Vide in it, and set to 183 F. Season eggplants with salt. Lay a vacuum-sealable bag on its side, make a layer of half the eggplant, spread one portion of tomato sauce, layer mozzarella, then parmesan, then cheese blend, then basil. Top with the second portion of tomato sauce.
2. Seal the bag carefully by the water displacement method, keeping it flat as possible. Submerge the bag flat in the water bath. Set the timer for 2 hours and cook. Release air 2 to 3 times within the first 30 minutes as eggplant releases gas as it cooks.
3. Once the timer has stopped, remove the bag gently and poke one corner of the bag using a pin to release liquid from the bag. Lay the bag flat on a serving plate, cut open the top of it and gently slide the lasagna onto the plate. Top with remaining tomato sauce, macadamia nuts, cheese blend, and Parmesan cheese. Melt and brown the cheese using a torch.

Balsamic Braised Cabbage Currants

Servings: 4
Cooking Time: 2 Hours
Ingredients:

- 1 and ½ pound, red cabbage
- ¼ cup, currants
- 1 thinly sliced shallot
- 3 thinly sliced garlic clove
- 1 tablespoon, balsamic vinegar
- 1 tablespoon, unsalted butter
- ½ teaspoon, kosher salt

Directions:

1. Prepare your Sous Vide water bath by dipping your immersion cooker and raising the temperature to 185ºF
2. Slice up your cabbage into quarters and remove the core
3. Chop up the cabbage into 1 and ½ inch pieces
4. Take 2 large sized heavy-duty zip bag and divide the cabbages between the bags
5. Divide the dry ingredients between the bags as well
6. Seal up the bags using immersion method
7. Submerge the bag underwater and let them cook for 2 hours
8. Once the cooking is done, remove the bag from the water and transfer it to a serving bowl
9. Add the juices
10. Season with some salt and vinegar and serve!

Nutrition Info: Per serving:Calories 204, Carbohydrates 9 g, Fats 16 g, Protein 6 g

VEGETABLES & SIDES

Chipotle & Black Beans

Servings: 6
Cooking Time: 6 Hours
Ingredients:
- 1 cup dry black beans
- 2 2/3 cup water
- 1/3 cup freshly squeezed orange juice
- 2 tablespoons orange zest
- 1 teaspoon salt
- 1 teaspoon cumin
- ½ teaspoon chipotle chili powder

Directions:
1. Prepare the Sous-vide water bath using your immersion circulator and raise the temperature to 193-degrees Fahrenheit.
2. Take a heavy-duty resealable plastic bag and add the listed ingredients into the bag.
3. Submerge it underwater and cook for 6 hours.
4. Once cooked, take the bag out from the water bath.
5. Pour the contents into a nice sauté pan and place it over medium heat.
6. Simmer until the amount has been reduced.
7. Once your desired texture is achieved, remove from the heat and serve!

Nutrition Info: Calories: 466 Carbohydrates: 15g Protein: 20g Fat: 37g Sugar: 3g Sodium: 546mg

Lightly Seasoned Beets

Cooking Time: 1½ Hours Cooking Temperature: 185°f
Ingredients:
- 12-16 small, fresh beets, trimmed, scrubbed and halved
- 2 tablespoons butter, softened
- 1/2 teaspoon salt
- 1/4 teaspoon freshly ground black pepper

Directions:
1. Attach the sous vide immersion circulator to a Cambro container or pot with water using an adjustable clamp and preheat water to 185°F.
2. Place beets in a single layer in a cooking pouch. Add butter, salt, and pepper. Seal pouch tightly after squeezing out the excess air. Place pouch in sous vide bath and set the cooking time for about 1½ hours.
3. Remove pouch from the sous vide bath and carefully open it.
4. Remove beets and serve immediately.

Pomme Purée

Servings: 4
Cooking Time: 30 Minutes
Ingredients:
- 1½ lb. potatoes, peeled
- 15-ounce vegan butter
- 8-ounce coconut milk
- A pinch of salt
- White pepper as needed

Directions:
1. Prepare your Sous-vide water bath using your immersion circulator and raise the temperature to 194-degrees Fahrenheit.
2. Slice the potatoes to 1 cm thick slices
3. Take your heavy-duty resealable zipper bag and add the potatoes, coconut milk, vegan butter and salt
4. Submerge underwater and let it cook for 30 minutes
5. Strain the mixture through a metal mesh/sieve and allow the butter mixture to pour into a bowl
6. Puree the potatoes by blending them or mashing them using a spoon
7. Pour the puree into the butter bowl
8. Season with pepper and serve!

Nutrition Info: Calories: 56 Carbohydrates: 2g Protein: 1g Fat: 5g Sugar: 0g Sodium: 56mg

Carrots With Butter

Cooking Time: 25 Mins Cooking Temperature: 185°f
Ingredients:
- Baby carrots
- Olive oil, as required
- Pinch of salt
- Butter, as required

Directions:

1. Attach the sous vide immersion circulator to a Cambro container or pot with water using an adjustable clamp and preheat water to 185°F.
2. Place carrots in a single layer in a cooking pouch. Add a little olive oil and salt. Seal pouch tightly after squeezing out the excess air. Place pouch in sous vide bath and set the cooking time for about 25 minutes.
3. Remove pouch from the sous vide bath and carefully open it. Remove carrots from pouch. With paper towels, pat dry carrots completely
4. Serve immediately with a topping of butter.

Pears In Pomegranate Juice

Servings: 8
Cooking Time: 30 Minutes
Ingredients:
- 8 pears
- 5 cups pomegranate juice
- ¾ cup sugar
- 1 cinnamon stick
- ¼ teaspoon nutmeg
- ¼ teaspoon ground cloves
- ¼ teaspoon allspice

Directions:
1. Preheat Sous Vide cooker to 176ºF.
2. Combine all ingredients, except the pears.
3. Simmer until the liquid is reduced by half.
4. Strain and place aside.
5. Gently scrub the pears or peel if desired.
6. Place each pear is sous Vide bag, and pour in some poaching liquid. Make sure each pear has the same level of poaching liquid.
7. Vacuum seal the pears and submerge in water.
8. Cook 30 minutes.
9. Open bags and remove pears carefully. Slice the pears and place onto a plate.
10. Cook the juices in a saucepan until thick.
11. Drizzle over pears.
12. Serve warm.

Nutrition Info: Per serving:Calories 243.5, Carbohydrates 59.4 g, Fats 0.3 g, Protein 0.8 g

Sous Vide Tomato Sauce

Servings: 4

Cooking Time: 15 Minutes
Ingredients:
- 4 cups cored and halved fresh tomatoes
- ½ onion, chopped
- ¼ cup fresh basil
- 2 garlic cloves, minced
- Salt to taste
- Freshly ground black pepper, to taste
- 5 tablespoons extra-virgin olive oil

Directions:
1. Prepare the Sous Vide water bath using your immersion circulator and raise the temperature to 176-degrees Fahrenheit.
2. Take a heavy-duty large resealable zip bag and add in the tomatoes, ¼ cup basil, garlic, onion, and oil. Seal using the immersion method.
3. Submerge it underwater and let it cook for 15 minutes.
4. Once cooked, transfer the contents to a blender and puree for about 1 minute.
5. Add a bit of salt and pepper and serve.

Nutrition Info: Calories: 117 Carbohydrates: 26g Protein: 5g Fat: 1g Sugar: 14g Sodium: 470mg

Acorn Squash

Cooking Time: 1 Hour Cooking Temperature: 194°f
Ingredients:
- 2 tablespoons butter
- Pinch of dried rosemary
- Pinch of salt
- 1 acorn squash, seeded and cut into wedges

Directions:
1. Attach the sous vide immersion circulator to a Cambro container or pot with water using an adjustable clamp and preheat water to 194°F.
2. In a pan, melt butter over medium heat until light brown specks appear, stirring occasionally. Stir in rosemary and salt and remove from heat.
3. Place acorn squash in a cooking pouch. Pour brown butter over squash wedges evenly. Seal pouch tightly after squeezing out the excess air. Place pouch in sous vide bath and set the cooking time for about 1 hour.

4. Remove pouch from the sous vide bath and carefully open it. Transfer squash wedges onto a serving platter and serve.

Strawberry Jam

Servings: 10
Cooking Time: 1 Hour 30 Minutes
Ingredients:
*   2 cups strawberries, coarsely chopped
*   1 cup white sugar
*   2 tbsp orange juice
Directions:
1. Put the ingredients into the vacuum bag and seal it.
2. Cook for 1 hour 30 minutes in the water bath, previously preheated to 180ºF.
3. Serve over ice cream or cheese cake, or store in the fridge in an airtight container.
Nutrition Info: Per serving:Calories 131, Carbohydrates 13 g, Fats 7 g, Protein 4 g

Beet Salad With Pecans

Servings: 4
Cooking Time: 1 Hour 5 Minutes
Ingredients:
*   1 ½ pounds beets, peeled and sliced 1/4-inch thick
*   1 medium-sized leek
*   2 garlic cloves, minced
*   1 cup baby arugula
*   1/4 cup mayonnaise
*   1 teaspoon grainy mustard
*   Salt and ground black pepper, to taste
*   1/3 teaspoon cumin seeds
*   2 teaspoons balsamic vinegar
*   1 tablespoon honey
*   1/4 cup pecan halves, roasted
Directions:
1. Preheat a sous vide water bath to 185 degrees F.
2. Place the beets in a cooking pouch; seal tightly.
3. Submerge the cooking pouch in the water bath; cook for 1 hour. Remove from the cooking pouch.
4. Add the leeks, garlic, and baby arugula; toss to combine.

5. Then, toss your salad with the mayo, mustard, salt, pepper, cumin, vinegar, and honey; toss again to combine well.
6. Serve topped with roasted pecan halves and enjoy!
Nutrition Info: 206 Calories; 7g Fat; 24g Carbs; 1g Protein; 12g Sugars

Potato Salad

Servings: 6
Cooking Time: 1 Hour 30 Minutes
Ingredients:
*   1 ½ pounds yellow potatoes or red potatoes
*   ½ cup chicken stock
*   Salt and pepper to taste
*   4 oz. thick cut bacon, sliced into about ¼-inch slices
*   ½ cup chopped onion
*   1/3 cup cider vinegar
*   4 scallions, thinly sliced
Directions:
1. Set Sous Vide cooker to 185ºF.
2. Cut potatoes in ¾-inch thick cubes.
3. Place potatoes and chicken stock to the zip-lock bag, making sure they are in a single layer; seal using immersion water method.
4. Place potatoes in a water bath and cook for 1 hour 30 minutes.
5. Meanwhile, in last 15 minutes heat non-stick skillet over medium-high heat. Add bacon and cook until crisp; remove bacon and add chopped onions. Cook until soften for 5-7 minutes.
6. Add vinegar and cook until reduced slightly.
7. Remove potatoes from the water bath and place them in skillet, with the cooking water.
8. Continue cooking for few minutes until liquid thickens.
9. Remove potatoes from the heat and stir in scallions; toss to combine.
10. Serve while still hot.
Nutrition Info: Per serving:Calories 108.8, Carbohydrates 19.9 g, Fats 1.6 g, Protein 3.7 g

Cardamom Apricots

Servings: 4
Cooking Time: 1 Hour
Ingredients:
- 1 pint small apricots, halved
- 1 tablespoon unsalted butter
- 1 teaspoon cardamom seeds, freshly ground
- ½ teaspoon ground ginger
- A pinch of smoked sea salt
- Fresh basil for garnishing, chopped

Directions:
1. Prepare your Sous Vide water bath by increasing the temperature to 180-degrees Fahrenheit using an immersion circulator
2. Put the butter, apricots, ginger, cardamom, and salt in a large, heavy-duty plastic bag, and mix them well
3. Carefully seal the bag using the immersion method and submerge it in the hot water
4. Let it cook for 60 minutes and remove the bag once done
5. Put the apricots in serving bowls
6. Garnish by topping it up with basil
7. Serve!

Nutrition Info: Per serving:Calories: 270 ;Carbohydrate: 60g ;Protein: 1g ;Fat: 0g ;Sugar: 49g ;Sodium: 33mg

Herby Braised Leeks

Servings: 4
Cooking Time: 40 Minutes
Ingredients:
- 1 pound leeks, discard outer leaves and halved lengthwise
- 1 cup vegetable stock
- 2 tablespoons sesame oil
- 2 garlic cloves, sliced
- 2 thyme sprigs
- Sea salt and ground black pepper, to taste

Directions:
1. Preheat a sous vide water bath to 185 degrees F.
2. Place all of the above ingredients in a cooking pouch; seal tightly.
3. Submerge the cooking pouch in the water bath; cook for 35 minutes.

4. Taste, adjust the seasonings and serve with mashed potatoes. Bon appétit!
Nutrition Info: 139 Calories; 2g Fat; 13g Carbs; 9g Protein; 8g Sugars

Spicy Summer Medley

Servings: 6
Cooking Time: 1 Hour 20 Minutes
Ingredients:
- 1 pound kabocha pumpkin, cut into wedges
- 1/2 pound eggplants, sliced
- 1/2 pound cabbage
- 4 tablespoons sesame oil
- 4 cloves garlic, minced
- 1 teaspoon fresh ginger, grated
- 2 shallots, peeled and cut into wedges
- 1 red bell pepper, seeded and thinly sliced
- 1 yellow bell pepper, seeded and thinly sliced
- 1 serrano pepper, seeded and thinly sliced
- 1/4 cup sake
- 1/4 cup water
- 2 tablespoons ketchup
- 2 ripe tomatoes, chopped
- Salt and ground black pepper, to taste
- 1/2 teaspoon cayenne pepper
- 2 tablespoons miso
- 2 teaspoons sugar

Directions:
1. Preheat a sous vide water bath to 183 degrees F.
2. Place kabocha pumpkin, eggplants, and cabbage in separate cooking pouches; add 1 tablespoon of sesame oil to each pouch; seal tightly.
3. Submerge the cooking pouches in the water bath; cook for 45 minutes.
4. When the timer goes off, remove the pouch with eggplants; reserve. Set the timer for a further 20 minutes.
5. Remove the pumpkin and cabbage from the cooking pouches; reserve.
6. Heat the remaining tablespoon of sesame oil in a pot over a moderate heat.
7. Now, sauté the garlic, ginger, shallots and peppers until just softened. Pour in sake to deglaze your pan. Add the water and bring the mixture to a rolling boil for 5 minutes.

8. Add the rest of above ingredients, including the reserved vegetables. Now, decrease the heat to low to maintain a simmer; simmer approximately 8 minutes to allow the flavors to develop.

9. Ladle into individual bowls and serve warm. Bon appétit!

Nutrition Info: 216 Calories; 9g Fat; 25g Carbs; 8g Protein; 11g Sugars

Cheesy Grits

Cooking Time: 3 Hours Cooking Temperature: 180°f

Ingredients:
- 1 cup old fashioned grits
- 3 cups vegetable broth
- 1 cup cream
- 2 tablespoons cold butter, cut into small pieces
- 4 ounces /1/4 pound cheddar cheese, grated, plus extra for garnish
- Salt and freshly ground black pepper, to taste
- Paprika for garnish

Directions:
1. Attach the sous vide immersion circulator to a Cambro container or pot with water using an adjustable clamp and preheat water to 180°F.
2. In a large bowl, add grits, broth, and cream and beat until well combined. Add butter and gently stir.
3. Place grits mixture in a cooking pouch. Seal pouch tightly after squeezing out the excess air. Place pouch in sous vide bath and set the cooking time for about 2-3 hours.
4. Remove pouch from the sous vide bath and carefully open it. Transfer grits into a bowl. Immediately, add cheese and beat until well combined. Stir in salt and black pepper.
5. Serve immediately with a sprinkling of extra cheese and paprika.

Green Beans & Mandarin Hazelnuts

Servings: 9
Cooking Time: 60 Minutes
Ingredients:
- 1 lb. green beans, trimmed
- 2 small mandarin oranges
- 2 tablespoons butter
- ½ teaspoon salt
- 2 oz. toasted hazelnuts

Directions:
1. Prepare the Sous Vide water bath using your immersion circulator and increase the temperature to 185-degrees Fahrenheit
2. Put the green beans, butter, and salt in a zip bag
3. Zest one of the mandarins into the bag and keep the other for later use
4. Cut the zested mandarin in half and squeeze the juice into the bag
5. Use the immersion method to seal the bag
6. Submerge and cook for 60 minutes
7. Pre-heat your oven to 400-degrees Fahrenheit and toast the hazelnuts for 7 minutes
8. Remove the skin and chop roughly
9. Serve by putting the beans on a platter and topping them up with a garnish of toasted hazelnut and the remaining mandarin zest

Nutrition Info: Calories: 520 Carbohydrate: 48g Protein: 40g Fat: 18g Sugar: 8g Sodium: 131mg

Biscuits

Cooking Time: 2 Hours Cooking Temperature: 195°f

Ingredients:
- 1 cup all-purpose flour
- ½ Teaspoon granulated sugar
- 1 teaspoon baking powder
- ¼ Teaspoon baking soda
- ¼ Teaspoon salt
- ½ Cup chilled buttermilk
- 4 tablespoons unsalted butter, melted

Directions:
1. Attach the sous vide immersion circulator to a Cambro container or pot with water using an adjustable clamp and preheat water to 195°F. Grease 5 half-pint canning jars generously.
2. In a medium bowl, mix together flour, sugar, baking powder, baking soda, and salt.
3. In another bowl, add buttermilk and butter and stir until butter forms distinct clumps in the buttermilk. Add buttermilk mixture into flour mixture and stir until just combined.
4. Divide dough between prepared jars evenly. With a damp towel, wipe off sides and tops of jars.

5.	Cover each jar with the lid just tight. /Do not over-tighten jars; air will need to escape. Place jars in sous vide bath and set the cooking time for about 2 hours.

6.	Remove the jars from the sous vide bath and carefully remove the lids. Place jars onto a wire rack to cool for about 5 minutes.

7.	Carefully remove biscuits from jars and serve warm.

Broccoli With Roasted Red Peppers

Cooking Time: 50 Minutes Cooking Temperature: 183°f

Ingredients:
- 2 canned roasted red peppers, rinse, seeded and cut into strips lengthwise
- 2 cups broccoli florets
- 1 garlic clove, minced
- ½ Teaspoon salt
- ¼ Teaspoon freshly ground black pepper
- 1 tablespoon butter
- ¼ cup Parmesan cheese, grated freshly

Directions:
1.	Attach the sous vide immersion circulator to a Cambro container or pot with water using an adjustable clamp and preheat water to 183°F.

2.	Place red pepper strips in a cooking pouch.

3.	In a bowl, mix together broccoli, garlic, salt, and black pepper. In another cooking pouch, place broccoli mixture and butter.

4.	Seal pouches tightly after squeezing out the excess air. Place the pouch of broccoli in sous vide bath and set the cooking time for about 30 minutes. After 10-15 minutes, add pouch of red peppers to the sous vide bath.

5.	Remove pouches from the sous vide bath and carefully open them. Remove vegetables from pouch and discard cooking liquid.

6.	Transfer vegetables into warm serving bowls evenly. Garnish with Parmesan cheese and serve immediately.

Ma Po Tofu

Servings: 6

Cooking Time: 90 Minutes

Ingredients:
- 1 cup vegetable broth
- 2 tablespoons tomato paste
- 1 tablespoon grated ginger
- 1 tablespoon rice wine vinegar
- 1 tablespoon agave nectar
- 2 teaspoons sriracha sauce
- 3 cloves minced garlic
- 1 teaspoon soy sauce
- 2 boxes cubed silken tofu

Directions:
1.	Prepare the Sous Vide water bath using your immersion circulator and increase the temperature to 185-degrees Fahrenheit

2.	Whisk all of the listed ingredients in a bowl, except the tofu

3.	Put the tofu in a zip bag and add the mixture

4.	Seal the bag using the immersion method and cook for 1½ hours

5.	Serve!

Nutrition Info: Calories: 560 Carbohydrate: 83g Protein: 33g Fat: 14g Sugar: 1g Sodium: 402mg

Wine Maple Poached Fruits

Servings: 4

Cooking Time: 1 Hour

Ingredients:
- 1 pound ripe peaches, peeled, pitted and halved
- 1 cup white wine
- 2 cups water
- 1 cup maple syrup
- 1 /1-inch piece fresh ginger, peeled
- 1 teaspoon whole cloves
- 1 vanilla pod
- 2 sticks cinnamon
- 1/3 cup almonds, blanched

Directions:
1.	Preheat a sous vide water bath to 170 degrees F.

2.	Place all ingredient, except for almonds, in a large-sized cooking pouch; seal tightly.

3.	Submerge the cooking pouch in the water bath; cook for 50 minutes.

4. Pour the cooking liquid into a pan that is preheated over a moderate flame. Bring to a rolling boil. Immediately turn the heat to medium.

5. Continue to cook an additional 6 minutes, or until the sauce is slightly thickened and syrupy.

6. To serve, arrange peach on a serving plate; spoon the wine/maple syrup over them; garnish with blanched almonds. Bon appétit!

Nutrition Info: 294 Calories; 3g Fat; 71g Carbs; 9g Protein; 64g Sugars

Easy Garden Green Beans

Servings: 4

Cooking Time: 45 Minutes

Ingredients:
- 1 ½ pounds fresh green beans, trimmed and snapped in half
- 2 tablespoons olive oil
- Flaky salt and lemon pepper, to taste
- 3 cloves garlic, minced

Directions:
1. Preheat a sous vide water bath to 183 degrees F.
2. Place the green beans, 1 tablespoon of olive oil, salt, and lemon pepper in a large cooking pouch; seal tightly.
3. Submerge the cooking pouch in the water bath; cook for 40 minutes.
4. In the meantime, heat the remaining tablespoon of olive oil in a pan; sauté the garlic for 1 minute or until aromatic.
5. Add the green beans to the pan with garlic, stir, and serve immediately. Enjoy!

Nutrition Info: 100 Calories; 6g Fat; 1g Carbs; 1g Protein; 4g Sugars

Crunchy Apple Salad With Almonds

Servings: 4

Cooking Time: 40 Minutes + Chilling Time

Ingredients:
- 3 crisp eating apples, cored, and sliced
- 2 tablespoons honey
- 1/2 cup dried cranberries
- 1 cup almonds
- 6 ounces package mixed spring greens

- 1/4 cup sour cream
- 1/4 cup mayonnaise
- 1 teaspoon yellow mustard
- 1/2 tablespoon lime juice
- 1 tablespoon sugar
- Salt and white pepper, to your liking

Directions:
1. Preheat a sous vide water bath to 160 degrees F.
2. Add the apples and honey to a cooking pouch; seal tightly.
3. Submerge the cooking pouches in the water bath; cook for 35 minutes. Remove the apples from the cooking pouch and let them cool completely.
4. Transfer the apples to a nice salad bowl. Add the cranberries, almonds, and greens.
5. In a mixing bowl, whisk the sour cream, mayonnaise, mustard, lime juice, sugar, salt, and pepper. Whisk until sugar is dissolved.
6. Dress the salad and serve well-chilled. Bon appétit!

Nutrition Info: 193 Calories; 9g Fat; 39g Carbs; 3g Protein; 28g Sugars

Chinese Black Bean Sauce

Servings: 4

Cooking Time: 90 Minutes

Ingredients:
- 4 cups halved green beans
- 3 minced garlic cloves
- 2 teaspoons rice wine vinegar
- 1½ tablespoons prepared black bean sauce
- 1 tablespoon olive oil

Directions:
1. Prepare the Sous-vide water bath using your immersion circulator and raise the temperature to 170-degrees Fahrenheit.
2. Add all the listed ingredients into a large mixing bowl alongside the green beans. Coat everything evenly.
3. Take a heavy-duty zip bag and add the mixture.
4. Zip the bag using the immersion method and submerge it underwater.
5. Cook for about 1 hour and 30 minutes.
6. Once cooked, take it out and serve immediately!

Nutrition Info: Calories: 375 Carbohydrates: 14g Protein: 12g Fat: 12g Sugar: 5g Sodium: 485mg

Honey Poached Pears

Servings: 2
Cooking Time: 45 Minutes
Ingredients:

- 1 pear, thinly sliced
- 1 lb. honey
- ½ cup of walnuts
- 4 tablespoons shaved Parmesan
- 2 cups rocket leaves
- Salt and pepper as needed
- 2 tablespoons lemon juice
- 2 tablespoons extra-virgin olive oil

Directions:

1. Prepare your water bath using your Sous Vide immersion circulator and raise the temperature to 158-degrees Fahrenheit
2. Put the honey, smeared pears in a heavy-duty resealable bag
3. Seal using the immersion method and submerge
4. Cook for 45 minutes
5. Put the contents of the bag in a bowl
6. Add the remaining dressing ingredients and toss well
7. Serve!

Nutrition Info: Calories: 189 Carbohydrate: 16g Protein: 9g Fat: 12g Sugar: 5g Sodium: 437mg

Bright Pea Mash

Servings: 4
Cooking Time: 45 Minutes
Ingredients:

- 1 pound green peas, frozen thawed
- 2 garlic cloves, smashed
- 2 tablespoons scallions
- 1/4 cup basil leaves
- 1 tablespoon fresh dill weed
- 1/2 stick butter
- 1/4 cup sour cream /10 % butterfat
- 2 tablespoons pecorino cheese, grated
- Sea salt flakes and ground black pepper to taste

Directions:

1. Preheat a sous vide water bath to 183 degrees F.
2. Add the peas, garlic, scallions, basil, and dill to cooking pouches; seal tightly.
3. Submerge the cooking pouches in the water bath; cook for 40 minutes.
4. Add the contents of cooking pouches to your food processor. Add the remaining ingredients and puree until creamy and uniform.
5. Taste, adjust the seasonings and serve. Bon appétit!

Nutrition Info: 196 Calories; 18g Fat; 14g Carbs; 4g Protein; 2g Sugars

Okra With Chili Yogurt

Servings: 6
Cooking Time: 1 Hour
Ingredients:

- 2.5lb. fresh okra
- 4 tablespoons olive oil
- 1 ½ tablespoon lime zest
- 2 cloves garlic, crushed
- Salt and white pepper, to taste
- Yogurt:
- 1 cup Greek yogurt
- 2 teaspoons chili powder
- ¼ cup chopped cilantro

Directions:

1. Preheat your Sous Vide to 178ºF.
2. Divide the fresh okra among two cooking bags.
3. Drizzle the okra with 2 ½ tablespoons olive oil (divided per bag), lime zest, and season to taste. Add one clove garlic per pouch.
4. Vacuum seal the bags and submerge in water.
5. Cook the okra 1 hour. Remove from a water bath and drain the accumulated liquid in a bowl. Place the okra in a separate bowl.
6. In a medium bowl, combine Greek yogurt, chili powder, cilantro, and accumulated okra water. Stir to combine.
7. Heat remaining olive oil in a skillet over medium-high heat.
8. Fry okra in the heated oil for 2 minutes.
9. Serve warm, with chili yogurt.

Nutrition Info: Per serving:Calories 189.3, Carbohydrates 16.5 g, Fats 10.5 g, Protein 7.2 g

Portobello Mushrooms With Grilled Vegetables

Servings: 4
Cooking Time: 1 Hour
Ingredients:
- 2 pounds Portobello mushrooms
- 2 tablespoons olive oil
- 1/2 tablespoon pear cider vinegar
- 2 garlic cloves, crushed
- Sea salt and freshly ground black pepper, to taste
- 1/2 teaspoon lemon thyme
- 1 teaspoon sage
- 1 teaspoon rosemary
- 1 teaspoon basil
- 1/2 teaspoon oregano
- 1 yellow summer squash, cut into 1/2-inch slices
- 1 red onion, cut into wedges

Directions:
1. Preheat a sous vide water bath to 140 degrees F.
2. Then, simply place all of the above ingredients, except for the summer squash and red onion, in cooking pouches; seal tightly.
3. Submerge the cooking pouches in the water bath; cook for 50 minutes.
4. In the meantime, place the summer squash and red onion on a grilling grid. Cover and grill vegetable over medium heat about 10 minutes or until crisp-tender.
5. Serve sous vide mushrooms with grilled vegetables on the side. Bon appétit!

Nutrition Info: 141 Calories; 1g Fat; 15g Carbs; 9g Protein; 4g Sugars

Honey Kumquats

Servings: 4
Cooking Time: 1 Hour
Ingredients:
- 1 lb. kumquats
- ¼ cup honey
- ¼ teaspoon kosher salt

Directions:
1. Prepare your Sous Vide water bath using your immersion circulator and raise the temperature to 194-degrees Fahrenheit
2. Slice your Kumquats into ⅛ inch thick slices, carefully remove the stems and de-seed them
3. Put the honey, kumquat, and salt in a heavy-duty, resealable bag and seal it using the immersion method/water displacement method
4. Submerge it in the hot water and cook for 60 minutes
5. Prepare an ice bath and put the bag in the bath
6. Cool and serve!

Nutrition Info: Per serving:Calories: 390 ;Carbohydrate: 28g ;Protein: 5g ;Fat: 30g ;Sugar: 23g ;Sodium: 118mg

Italian-style Fruit Toast

Servings: 6
Cooking Time: 1 Hour 20 Minutes
Ingredients:
- 1 ½ cups granulated sugar
- 1 ½ cups water
- 2 tablespoons fresh cilantro, chiffonade
- 2 tablespoons freshly squeezed orange juice
- 1 cup banana, sliced
- 1 cup cherries
- 1 cup pears, cored and sliced
- 2 tablespoons coconut oil, melted
- 1/2 teaspoon pure vanilla extract
- 1/4 cup honey
- 8 slices ciabatta, cut on the bias
- 1 cup ricotta, at room temperature
- 1/4 teaspoon ground cinnamon

Directions:
1. In a saucepan, cook the sugar, water, cilantro, and orange juice over medium-low heat; allow it to simmer about 8 minutes.
2. Preheat a sous vide water bath to 183 degrees F.
3. Separate fruits in individual cooking pouches by type; divide the prepared syrup among cooking pouches, seal tightly, and let it sit for 30 minutes.
4. Submerge the cooking pouches in the water bath; cook for 15 minutes.

5. Remove the pouches with banana and cherries from the water bath and reserve the liquid. Cook the pears an additional 25 minutes.

6. Toss the sous vide fruit with coconut oil, vanilla extract, and honey. Serve on ciabatta slices topped with the reserved syrup, ricotta and ground cinnamon. Bon appétit!

Nutrition Info: 282 Calories; 2g Fat; 49g Carbs; 8g Protein; 37g Sugars

Parsnips

Cooking Time: 1 Hour 40 Mins Cooking Temperature: 185°f

Ingredients:

- Vegetable broth, enough to cover parsnips in cooking bag
- 2-3 parsnips, peeled and cut into thick rounds
- 2-3 teaspoons fresh thyme leaves
- Butter, as required

Directions:

1. Attach the sous vide immersion circulator to a Cambro container or pot with water using an adjustable clamp and preheat water to 185°F.

2. In a cooking pouch, place parsnip rounds, thyme, and enough broth to cover. Seal pouch tightly after squeezing out the excess air. Place pouch in sous vide bath and set the cooking time for about 45 minutes and no more than 90 minutes.

3. Remove pouch from the sous vide bath and carefully open it. Remove parsnips from pouch, reserving broth in a bowl. With paper towels, pat dry parsnip rounds completely.

4. In a non-stick frying pan, melt butter over high heat and cook parsnip rounds until browned on both sides.

5. Add reserved broth with some water over high heat and cook until sauce becomes thick, basting parsnips occasionally with sauce.

6. Serve parsnips with pan sauce.

Garlic & Paprika Sweet Potatoes

Cooking Time: 1 Hour Cooking Temperature: 185°f

Ingredients:

- 7 tablespoons salted butter, softened

- 4½ tablespoons maple syrup
- 10 roasted, smoked garlic cloves
- 2 teaspoons fresh thyme, chopped
- 2 teaspoons smoked paprika
- Sea salt, to taste
- 2 pounds /1 kg sweet potatoes, peeled and chopped

Directions:

1. Attach the sous vide immersion circulator to a Cambro container or pot with water using an adjustable clamp and preheat water to 185°F.

2. In a bowl, add all ingredients except sweet potatoes and mix until well combined.

3. Place sweet potatoes and butter mixture in a cooking pouch. Seal pouch tightly after squeezing out the excess air. Place pouch in sous vide bath and set the cooking time for about 45-60 minutes.

4. Remove pouch from the sous vide bath and carefully open it. Remove sweet potatoes from pouch.

5. Heat a sauté pan and cook sweet potatoes until golden brown.

Ratatouille

Cooking Time: 1 Hour Cooking Temperature: 176°f

Ingredients:

- 1 pound Japanese eggplants, halved lengthwise
- ½ Pound zucchini, halved lengthwise
- ½ Pound yellow squash, halved lengthwise
- 1 red bell pepper, seeded and cut into quarters
- 5 tablespoons extra-virgin olive oil, divided
- Salt and freshly ground black pepper, to taste
- 1 Spanish onion, cut in ½-inch pieces
- 3 garlic cloves, minced
- 1 teaspoon red pepper flakes
- ½ Pound plum tomatoes, peeled and roughly chopped
- ½ Cup dry white wine
- 1 teaspoon thyme leaves
- 2 tablespoons fresh parsley, chopped
- ½ Cup fresh basil leaves

Directions:

1. Attach the sous vide immersion circulator to a Cambro container or pot with water using an adjustable clamp and preheat water to 176°F.

2. In a large bowl, add eggplant, zucchini, squash, bell pepper, 3 tablespoons of oil, salt, and black pepper and toss to coat well.

3. Heat a large skillet over medium-high heat and sear vegetable mixture in batches for about 4 minutes per side. Transfer vegetable mixture back into the bowl.

4. In the same skillet, add 1 tablespoon of olive oil over medium-high heat and sauté onion for about 8 minutes. Add garlic and red pepper flakes and sauté for about 1 more minute.

5. Stir in tomatoes and cook for about 1 minute. Add white wine, bring to a boil, and cook for about 1 minute. Remove from heat and stir in thyme.

6. Cut all cooked vegetables into ½-inch pieces. Add vegetable mixture into tomato mixture and stir to combine.

7. Place vegetable mixture in a cooking pouch. Seal pouch tightly after squeezing out the excess air. Place pouch in sous vide bath and set the cooking time for about 40 minutes.

8. Remove pouch from the sous vide bath and carefully open it. Transfer vegetable mixture into a large serving bowl. Stir in parsley and drizzle with remaining oil.

9. Garnish with basil and serve.

Colorful Veggies With Tomato Sorbet

Servings: 4
Cooking Time: 12 Minutes
Ingredients:
- 8 carrots, halved
- 12 spears green asparagus
- 1 cup fresh peas
- 3 tablespoons olive oil
- Salt and pepper, to taste
- Sorbet:
- ¼ cup water
- 2 tablespoons sugar
- 4 ripe tomatoes, peeled
- 2 tablespoons fresh lemon juice
- 1 tablespoon tomato paste
- Salt and black pepper, to taste

Directions:

1. Make the sorbet; in a food blender, blend the tomatoes until pureed.

2. Bring water, sugar, and basil to a boil in a saucepan. Remove from heat and allow to cool. Pour in the tomatoes and add tomato paste. Stir to combine. Season to taste with salt and pepper.

3. Place the sorbet into a freezer. Freeze 2-4 hours or until firm.

4. Make the vegetables; peel and trim asparagus.

5. Place the asparagus in one Souse vide bag and add 1 tablespoon olive oil.

6. In a separate bag, place carrots and peas. Drizzle with olive oil. Vacuum seal both bags.

7. Set the Sous Vide to 190ºF.

8. Cook the carrots and peas 12 minutes in heated water. After the carrots have been cooked 8 minutes, add asparagus.

9. Remove the bags from Sous Vide. Unpack the bags and arrange veggies onto a serving plate. Season to taste.

10. Serve veggies with a scoop of tomato sorbet.

Nutrition Info: Per serving:Calories 243.4, Carbohydrates 30.8 g, Fats 11 g, Protein 5.3 g

Brussels Sprouts With Garlic

Cooking Time: 1 Hour Cooking Temperature: 180°f
Ingredients:
- 1 tablespoon olive oil
- 2 garlic cloves, smashed and minced
- Pinch of salt
- Freshly ground black pepper, to taste
- 1 pound Brussels sprouts, trimmed

Directions:

1. Attach the sous vide immersion circulator to a Cambro container or pot with water using an adjustable clamp and preheat water to 180°F.

2. In a bowl, add all ingredients except Brussels sprouts and mix until well combined.

3. Place Brussels sprouts and oil mixture in a cooking pouch. Seal pouch tightly after squeezing out the excess air. Place pouch in sous vide bath and set the cooking time for about 1 hour.

4. Preheat a grill to medium heat.

5. Remove pouch from the sous vide bath and carefully open it. Remove Brussels sprouts from pouch.

6. Thread Brussels sprouts onto pre-soaked bamboo skewers. Grill for about 2-3 minutes per side.

Sous Vide Garlic Tomatoes

Servings: 4
Cooking Time: 45 Minutes
Ingredients:
- 4 pieces cored and diced tomatoes
- 2 tablespoons extra-virgin olive oil
- 3 minced garlic cloves
- 1 teaspoon dried oregano
- 1 teaspoon fine sea salt

Directions:
1. Prepare the Sous-vide water bath using your immersion circulator and raise the temperature to 145-degrees Fahrenheit.
2. Add all the listed ingredients to the resealable bag and seal using the immersion method.
3. Submerge underwater and let it cook for 45 minutes.
4. Once cooked, transfer the tomatoes to a serving plate.
5. Serve with some vegan French bread slices.
Nutrition Info: Calories: 289 Carbohydrates: 44g Protein: 11g Fat: 8g Sugar: 2g Sodium: 326mg

Taiwanese Corn

Cooking Time: 22 Mins Cooking Temperature: 185°f
Ingredients:
- 3 ears of summer corn
- 3 garlic cloves
- 1 stalk scallion, chopped roughly
- 2 tablespoons butter
- 3 tablespoons dark soy sauce
- 2 tablespoons chili sauce
- 1 tablespoon sugar
- Salt, to taste

Directions:
1. Attach the sous vide immersion circulator to a Cambro container or pot with water using an adjustable clamp and preheat water to 185°F.

2. In a food processor, add all ingredients except corn and salt and pulse until smooth.
3. Place corn and butter mixture in a cooking pouch. Seal pouch tightly after squeezing out the excess air. Place pouch in sous vide bath and set the cooking time for about 20 minutes.
4. Preheat the broiler of oven to high.
5. Remove pouch from the sous vide bath carefully open it. Remove corn ears from pouch.
6. Arrange corn ears onto a baking sheet and broil for about 2 minutes. Serve immediately.

Squash Casseroles

Servings: 4
Cooking Time: 1 Hour
Ingredients:
- 2 tablespoons unsalted butter
- ¾ cup onion, chopped
- 1½ lbs. zucchini, quartered lengthwise and sliced into ¼ inch thick pieces
- Kosher salt as needed
- Ground black pepper as needed
- ½ cup whole milk
- 2 large whole eggs
- ½ cup crumbled plain potato chips for serving

Directions:
1. Prepare your water bath using your Sous Vide immersion circulator and raise the temperature to 176-degrees Fahrenheit
2. Take 4 x 1-pint canning jars and grease them
3. Take a large skillet and put it over medium heat. Add the butter, melt the butter
4. Add the onions and sauté for 7 minutes
5. Add the zucchini and sauté for 10 minutes and season with pepper and salt
6. Divide the zucchini mix into the greased jars and allow them to cool
7. Whisk the milk, salt, and eggs in a bowl
8. Grind some pepper and mix well
9. Divide the mixture amongst the jars and place the lids loosely on top
10. Submerge underwater and cook for 60 minutes
11. Allow to cool for few minutes and serve over potato chips

Nutrition Info: Per serving:Calories: 319 ;Carbohydrate: 29g ;Protein: 10g ;Fat: 19g ;Sugar: 3g ;Sodium: 539mg

Pickle In A Jar

Servings: 6
Cooking Time: 15 Minutes
Ingredients:
- 1 cup white wine vinegar
- ½ cup beet sugar
- 2 teaspoons kosher salt
- 1 tablespoon pickling spice
- 2 English cucumbers sliced up into ¼ inch thick slices
- ½ white onion, thinly sliced

Directions:
1. Prepare the Sous-vide water bath using your immersion circulator and raise the temperature to 180-degrees Fahrenheit.
2. Take a large bowl and add the vinegar, sugar, salt, pickling spice and whisk them well.
3. Transfer to a heavy-duty resealable zipper bag alongside the cucumber and sliced onions and seal using the immersion method.
4. Submerge underwater and let it cook for 15 minutes.
5. Transfer the bag to an ice bath
6. Pour the mixture into a 4-6 ounce mason jar
7. Serve or store!

Nutrition Info: Calories: 117 Carbohydrates: 27g Protein: 1g Fat: 1g Sugar: 19g Sodium: 304mg

Queso Blanco Dip

Cooking Time: 30 Mins Cooking Temperature: 175°f
Ingredients:
- 1½ cups Asadero or Chihuahua cheese, shredded finely
- ¼ Cup half-and-half cream
- 4 ounces /1/4 pound green chilies, chopped
- 1 Serrano pepper, stemmed and chopped finely
- 2 tablespoons onion, grated
- 2 teaspoons ground cumin
- ½ Teaspoon salt

Directions:

1. Attach the sous vide immersion circulator to a Cambro container or pot with water using an adjustable clamp and preheat water to 175°F.
2. Place all ingredients except bread in a cooking pouch. Seal pouch tightly after squeezing out the excess air. Place pouch in sous vide bath and set the cooking time for about 30 minutes. Remove pouch from bath occasionally and massage mixture to mix.
3. Remove the pouch from the sous vide bath and carefully open it. Immediately, transfer dip into a bowl and serve.

Mashed Potato

Servings: 4
Cooking Time: 1 Hour
Ingredients:
- 1 lb. russet potatoes, peeled and sliced
- 8 tablespoons butter
- ½ cup heavy cream
- 1 teaspoon kosher salt

Directions:
1. Prepare your water bath using your Sous Vide immersion circulator and raise the temperature to 190-degrees Fahrenheit
2. Add the heavy cream, russet potatoes, kosher salt, and butter into a heavy-duty zip bag and seal using the immersion method
3. Submerge and cook for 60 minutes
4. Pass the contents through a food processor into a large bowl
5. Mix them well and serve!

Nutrition Info: Per serving:Calories: 226 ;Carbohydrate: 34g ;Protein: 5g ;Fat: 7g ;Sugar: 3g ;Sodium: 93mg

Corn On The Cob

Cooking Time: 30 Mins Cooking Temperature: 183°f
Ingredients:
- 4 ears corn, in the husk, both ends trimmed
- 2 tablespoons butter, plus extra for serving
- Kosher salt, to taste
- Fresh cilantro, chopped, as required
- Garlic cloves, minced, as required

Directions:

1. Attach the sous vide immersion circulator to a Cambro container or pot with water using an adjustable clamp and preheat water to 183°F.
2. In 2 cooking pouches, divide all ingredients evenly. Seal pouch tightly after squeezing out the excess air. Place pouches in sous vide bath and set the cooking time for about 30 minutes.
3. Remove pouches from the sous vide bath and carefully open them. Remove corn ears from pouches.
4. Carefully, remove corn from husks. Discard husks.
5. Serve corn with extra butter.

7. Stir in the pepper flakes and parsley
8. Take a large liquid measuring cup and whisk in eggs and milk, season the mix with salt
9. Divide the egg mixture amongst the jars together with the vegetables
10. Wipe off the tops, using a damp cloth, and tighten the lids using the fingertip method
11. Place the jars in your water bath and cook them for 60 minutes
12. Once done, remove the jars from your water bath and remove the lids
13. Allow to cool and serve!

Nutrition Info: Calories: 465 Carbohydrate: 34g Protein: 29g Fat: 23g Sugar: 5g Sodium: 516mg

Vegetable Frittata

Servings: 5
Cooking Time: 1 Hour
Ingredients:
- 1 tablespoon extra-virgin olive oil
- 1 medium onion, chopped
- Kosher salt as needed
- 4 cloves garlic, minced
- 1 small rutabaga, peeled and diced
- 2 medium-sized carrots, peeled and diced
- 1 medium-sized parsnip, peeled and diced
- 1 cup butternut squash, peeled and diced
- 6 oz. oyster mushrooms, roughly chopped and trimmed
- ¼ cup fresh parsley leaves, minced
- A pinch of red pepper flakes
- 5 large whole eggs
- ¼ cup whole milk

Directions:
1. Prepare your Sous Vide water bath using your immersion circulator and raise the temperature to 176-degrees Fahrenheit
2. Grease your canning jars with oil
3. Take a large-sized skillet and add the oil in it and place over a medium high heat
4. Add your onions to the heated skillet, stir cook for about 5 minutes, season with some salt
5. Add the garlic and stir cook for few more minutes
6. Add the carrots, rutabaga, mushrooms, butternut squash and parsnips, season with some salt and cook for 10-15 more minutes

Stuffed Apples

Servings: 4
Cooking Time: 90 Minutes
Ingredients:
- 4 golden apples
- ¼ cup palm sugar + 1 ½ tablespoons
- 1 tablespoon chopped dates
- 3 tablespoons raisins
- 2 tablespoons butter
- ¼ teaspoon cinnamon
- 1/3 cup organic apple juice
- 1 ½ tablespoons whipping cream
- To garnish:
- A handful of chopped walnuts

Directions:
1. Preheat your Sous Vide cooker to 185ºF.
2. Core the apples, leaving the bottom intact.
3. In a bowl, combine sugar, raisins, dates, butter, and cinnamon.
4. Fill the apples with prepared mixture.
5. Place each apple in Sous Vide bag and vacuum seal.
6. Cook the apples 90 minutes.
7. Combine the remaining sugar with apple juice in a saucepan.
8. Simmer until sauce is thick, for 10 minutes. Stir in the whipping cream.
9. Remove the apples from bags and serve on a plate.
10. Drizzle with sauce and sprinkle with walnuts.

Nutrition Info: Per serving: Calories 153.2, Carbohydrates 20.7 g, Fats 7.6 g, Protein 0.5 g

Red Onions Balsamic Glaze

Servings: 1
Cooking Time: 90 Minutes
Ingredients:
- 3 medium-sized red onions
- 1 tablespoon unsalted butter
- Salt and pepper as needed
- 2 tablespoons balsamic vinegar
- 1 tablespoon honey
- 2 teaspoons of fresh thyme leaves

Directions:
1. Prepare the Sous Vide water bath using your immersion circulator and raise the temperature to 185-degrees Fahrenheit
2. Peel the skin of the onion, making sure to keep the roots intact
3. Cut the onion into wedges through the root end
4. Put a large skillet over a medium/high heat
5. Add the butter and allow to heat up and melt
6. Add the onion and season with pepper and salt, cook for about 10 minutes until nicely browned
7. Put the balsamic vinegar and simmer on low heat for 1 minute
8. Remove from the heat and carefully stir in the honey
9. Transfer the onions to a large, heavy-duty zipper bag
10. Seal the bag using the immersion method and submerge
11. Cook for 90 minutes
12. Once done, remove from the water and arrange the onions on a serving plate
13. Sprinkle with fresh thyme and serve with pizza or a sandwich

Nutrition Info: Calories: 141 Carbohydrate: 19g Protein: 5g Fat: 6g Sugar: 6g Sodium: 87mg

Pear & Walnut Salad

Servings: 4
Cooking Time: 30 Minutes
Ingredients:
- 2 tablespoons honey
- 2 pears, cored, halved and thinly sliced
- ½ cup walnuts, lightly toasted and roughly chopped
- ½ cup shaved parmesan
- 4 cups arugula
- Sea salt and pepper as needed
- Garlic Dijon Dressing
- ¼ cup olive oil
- 1 tablespoon white wine vinegar
- 1 teaspoon Dijon mustard
- 1 garlic clove, minced
- Salt as needed

Directions:
1. Prepare your Sous Vide water bath using your immersion circulator and raise the temperature to 159-degrees Fahrenheit
2. Put the honey in a heat-proof bowl
3. Heat for 20 seconds
4. Put the pears in the honey and mix well
5. Put them in a heavy-duty resealable bag and seal using the immersion method
6. Cook for 30 minutes and plunge the bag into an ice water bath for 5 minutes
7. Chill in your fridge for 3 hours
8. Add all of the dressing ingredients and give the jar a nice shake
9. Leave it in your fridge for a while
10. Serve by placing the walnuts, arugula, and parmesan in a large bowl
11. Add your drained pear slices and the dressing
12. Toss everything well and season with pepper and salt

Nutrition Info: Calories: 377 Carbohydrate: 56g Protein: 5g Fat: 14g Sugar: 35g Sodium: 165mg

POULTRY RECIPES

Caesar Salad Tortilla Rolls With Turkey

Servings: 4
Cooking Time: 1 Hour 40 Minutes
Ingredients:

- 2 garlic cloves, minced
- 2 skinless, boneless turkey breasts
- Salt and black pepper to taste
- 1 cup mayonnaise
- 2 tbsp freshly squeezed lemon juice
- 1 tsp anchovy paste
- 1 tsp Dijon mustard
- 1 tsp soy sauce
- 4 cups iceberg lettuce
- 4 tortillas

Directions:

1.   Prepare a water bath and place the Sous Vide in it. Set to 152 F. Season the turkey breast with salt and pepper and put in a vacuum-sealable bag. Release air by the water displacement method, seal and submerge the bag in the water bath. Cook for 1 hour and 30 minutes.

2.   Combine the mayonnaise, garlic, lemon juice, anchovy paste, mustard, soy sauce, and remaining salt and pepper. Allow to rest in the fridge. Once the timer has stopped, remove the turkey and pat dry. Slice the turkey. Mix the lettuce with the cold dressing. Pour one-quarter of the turkey mixture into each tortilla and fold. Cut by the half and serve with the dressing.

Chicken & Avocado Salad

Servings: 2
Cooking Time: 75 Minutes
Ingredients:

- 1 chicken breast
- 1 avocado, sliced
- 10 pieces of halved cherry tomatoes
- 2 cups chopped lettuce
- 2 tablespoons olive oil
- 1 tablespoon lemon juice
- 1 garlic clove, crushed
- Salt and pepper as needed
- 2 teaspoons honey

Directions:

1.   Prepare your Sous Vide water bath, using your immersion circulator, and raise the temperature to 140-degrees Fahrenheit

2.   Add the breast to a Sous Vide zip bag and seal using the immersion method, submerge and cook for 75 minutes

3.   Season the breast with salt and pepper

4.   Pan fry 1 tablespoon of olive oil for 30 seconds

5.   Slice the breasts

6.   Add the garlic, lemon juice, honey and olive oil in a small bowl

7.   Add the lettuce, cherry tomatoes and avocado and toss

8.   Top the salad with chicken and season with pepper and salt

9.   Serve!

Nutrition Info: Calories: 520 Carbohydrate: 13g Protein: 68g Fat: 22g Sugar: 5g Sodium: 214mg

Teriyaki Chicken

Cooking Time: 56 Minutes Cooking Temperature: 145°f
Ingredients:

- For Chicken Bowl:
- 1 teaspoon garlic, minced
- 1 teaspoon fresh ginger, minced
- 4 tablespoons sake
- 4 tablespoons soy sauce
- 2 tablespoons rice wine vinegar
- 1 tablespoon brown sugar
- ¼ teaspoon chili powder
- Freshly ground black pepper, to taste
- 4 medium chicken thighs
- Salt, to taste
- 1 tablespoon corn flour
- 1 tablespoon water
- 4 eggs
- 2 cups white rice
- For Pickled Veggies:
- 3 cups veggies (2-parts carrot and cucumber, 1-part red onion and daikon), sliced finely
- 1 cup water
- 1 cup vinegar

- 2 tablespoons brown sugar
- 1 tablespoon salt

Directions:

1. Attach the sous vide immersion circulator to a Cambro container or pot with water using an adjustable clamp and preheat water to 145°F.
2. In a bowl, add garlic, ginger, sake, soy sauce, vinegar, brown sugar, chili powder, and black pepper and mix until well combined.
3. Place chicken thighs in a cooking pouch with the ginger mixture. Seal pouch tightly after removing the excess air. Place pouch in sous vide bath and set the cooking time for 50 minutes.
4. Gently place the eggs in the same sous vide bath for 50 minutes.
5. Prepare white rice according to the package's directions
6. For pickled veggies: add all ingredients in a pan over high heat and bring to a boil. Remove from heat and set aside until chicken cooks, keeping the pan covered.
7. Remove pouch and eggs from the sous vide bath. Carefully open pouch and remove chicken thighs, reserving the cooking liquid in a bowl. Pat dry chicken thighs with paper towels. Lightly season chicken thighs with salt.
8. In a small bowl, dissolve corn flour into water. Add the flour mixture to the bowl of reserved cooking liquid and stir to combine.
9. Heat a non-stick skillet over medium heat and sear chicken thighs for 2 minutes on each side. Add reserved liquid mixture to the skillet for the last minute of cooking and toss chicken thighs to coat.
10. With a slotted spoon, transfer chicken thighs to a platter. Continue cooking sauce in the skillet, stirring continuously, until it reaches desired thickness. Remove sauce from heat.
11. Drain pickled veggies and cut chicken thighs into desired slices.
12. Divide cooked rice into serving bowls and top with chicken slices. Pour sauce over chicken slices and place pickled veggies on the side. Crack the egg over rice and chicken. Season with salt and pepper and serve.

Duck Leg Confit

Servings: 2
Cooking Time: 12 Hours 10 Minutes
Ingredients:

- 2 duck legs
- 1 tbsp dried thyme
- 2 big bay leaves, crushed
- 6 tbsp duck fat
- Salt and pepper to taste
- Cranberry sauce for serving

Directions:

1. Preheat your Sous Vide machine to 167ºF.
2. Mix the bay leaves with salt, pepper and thyme, and season the duck legs with the mixture.
3. Refrigerate overnight.
4. In the morning, rinse the legs with cold water and carefully put them into the vacuum bag.
5. Add 4 tbsp duck fat, seal the bag removing the air as much as possible, put it into the water bath and set the cooking time for 12 hours.
6. Before serving, roast the legs in 2 remaining tbsp of duck fat until crispy.
7. Serve with cranberry sauce.

Nutrition Info: Per serving:Calories 529, Carbohydrates 15 g, Fats 37 g, Protein 34 g,

Sage Infused Turkey

Servings: 4-6
Cooking Time: 12 Hours
Ingredients:

- 2 turkey legs and thighs, with bone and skin
- 1 lemon, sliced
- 10 sage leaves
- 4 cloves garlic, halved
- Salt, to taste
- 1 teaspoon black peppercorns

Directions:

1. Preheat Sous Vide water bath to 148F.
2. Season the turkey with salt and place in a Sous Vide bag.
3. Add the lemon slices, sage, garlic, and peppercorns.
4. Vacuum seal the bag and cook the turkey 12 hours.
5. Finishing steps:

6. Remove the turkey from the bag and pat dry.
7. Heat non-stick skillet over medium-high heat.
8. Sear the turkey until golden-brown.
9. Serve warm.

Nutrition Info: Calories 310 Total Fat 4g Total Carb 6g Dietary Fiber 7g Protein 59g

Chili Chicken & Chorizo Tacos With Cheese

Servings: 8
Cooking Time: 3 Hours 25 Minutes
Ingredients:
- 2 pork sausages, castings removed
- 1 poblano pepper, stemmed and seeded
- ½ jalapeño pepper, stemmed and seeded
- 4 scallions, chopped
- 1 bunch fresh cilantro leaves
- ½ cup chopped fresh parsley
- 3 garlic cloves
- 2 tbsp lime juice
- 1 tsp salt
- ¾ tsp ground coriander
- ¾ tsp ground cumin
- 4 skinless, boneless chicken breasts, sliced
- 1 tbsp vegetable oil
- ½ yellow onion, sliced thinly
- 8 corn taco shells
- 3 tbsp Provolone cheese
- 1 tomato
- 1 Iceberg lettuce, shredded

Directions:
1. Put the ½ cup water, poblano pepper, jalapeño pepper, scallions, cilantro, parsley, garlic, lime juice, salt, coriander, and cumin in a blender and mix until smooth. Place the chicken strips and pepper mixture in a vacuum-sealable bag. Transfer to the fridge and allow to chill for 1 hour.
2. Prepare a water bath and place Sous Vide in it. Set to 141 F. Place the chicken mix in the bath. Cook for 1 hour and 30 minutes.
3. Heat oil in a skillet over medium heat and sauté onion for 3 minutes. Add in chorizo and cook for 5-7 minutes. Once the timer has stopped, remove the chicken. Discard cooking juices. Add in chicken and mix well. Fill the tortillas with chicken-chorizo mixture. Top with cheese, tomato and lettuce. Serve.

Chicken Thighs With Herbs

Servings: 4
Cooking Time: 4 Hours 10 Minutes
Ingredients:
- 1 pound chicken thighs
- 1 cup extra virgin olive oil
- ¼ cup apple cider vinegar
- 3 garlic cloves, crushed
- ½ cup freshly squeezed lemon juice
- 1 tbsp fresh basil, chopped
- 2 tbsp fresh thyme, chopped
- 1 tbsp fresh rosemary, chopped
- 1 tsp cayenne pepper
- 1 tsp salt

Directions:
1. Rinse the meat under cold running water and place in a large colander to drain. Set aside.
2. In a large bowl, combine olive oil with apple cider vinegar, garlic, lemon juice, basil, thyme, rosemary, salt, and cayenne pepper. Submerge thighs into this mixture and refrigerate for one hour. Remove the meat from the marinade and drain. Place in a large vacuum-sealable bag and cook en Sous Vide for 3 hours at 149 F.

Waldorf Chicken Salad

Servings: 4
Cooking Time: 120 Minutes
Ingredients:
- 2 skinless chicken breasts, boneless
- ½ teaspoon ground black pepper
- 1 tablespoon corn oil
- 1 Granny Smith apple, cored and diced
- 1 teaspoon lime juice
- ½ cup red grapes, cut in half
- 1 stick rib celery, diced
- 1/3 cup mayonnaise
- 2 teaspoons Chardonnay wine
- 1 teaspoon Dijon mustard
- 1 tablespoon kosher salt
- 1 Romaine lettuce head
- ½ cup walnuts, toasted and chopped

Directions:

1. Prepare your water bath using your Sous Vide immersion circulator, and increase the temperature to 145-degrees Fahrenheit
2. Take the chicken and season it with black pepper and salt. Put the seasoned chicken breast and corn oil in a large, resealable bag and seal using the immersion method
3. Cook for 2 hours and then remove the bag
4. Put the apple slices in a large-sized bowl, add the lime juice, and toss them well.
5. Add the celery and red grapes and stir well
6. Put the mayonnaise, Dijon mustard, and Chardonnay wine in a small bowl and mix well
7. Pour the whole mixture over the fruits and give them a nice toss
8. Remove the chicken breast from the plastic bag and discard the liquid
9. Dice the breast and place in a medium-sized bowl
10. Add some kosher salt and toss well
11. Put the seasoned chicken in with the rest of the salad and toss well
12. Dived your romaine lettuce amongst the salad bowls, spoon the salad on top of the lettuce, and garnish with some walnuts
13. Serve!

Nutrition Info: Per serving:Calories: 304 ;Carbohydrate: 34g ;Protein: 22g ;Fat: 9g ;Sugar: 7g ;Sodium: 529mg

Thyme Chicken With Lemon

Servings: 3
Cooking Time: 2 Hours 15 Minutes
Ingredients:

- 3 chicken thighs
- Salt and black pepper to taste
- 3 slices lemon
- 3 sprigs thyme
- 3 tbsp olive oil for searing

Directions:

1. Make a water bath, place Sous Vide in it, and set to 165 F. Season the chicken with salt and pepper. Top with lemon slices and thyme sprigs. Place them in a vacuum-sealable bag, release air by the water displacement method and seal the bag. Submerge in the water bag and set the timer for 2 hours.
2. Once the timer has stopped, remove and unseal the bag. Heat olive oil in a cast iron pan over high heat. Place the chicken thighs, skin down in the skillet and sear until golden brown.Garnish with extra lemon wedges. Serve with a side of cauli rice.

Buffalo Chicken Wings

Servings: 6
Cooking Time: 1 Hour And 20 Minutes
Ingredients:

- 3 lb chicken wings
- 3 tsp salt
- 2 tsp grounded garlic
- 2 tbsp smoked paprika
- 1 tsp sugar
- ½ cup hot sauce
- 5 tbsp butter
- 2 ½ cups almond flour
- Olive oil for frying

Directions:

1. Make a water bath, place Sous Vide in it, and set to 144 F.
2. Combine the wings, garlic, salt, sugar and smoked paprika. Coat the chicken evenly. Place in a sizable vacuum-sealable bag, release air by the water displacement method and seal the bag.
3. Submerge in the water. Set the timer to cook for 1 hour. Once the timer has stopped, remove and unseal the bag. Pour flour into a large bowl, add in chicken and toss to coat.
4. Heat oil in a pan over medium heat, fry the chicken until golden brown. Remove and set aside. In another pan, melt butter and add the hot sauce. Coat the wings with butter and hot sauce. Serve as an appetizer

Honey Flavored Chicken Wings

Servings: 2
Cooking Time: 135 Minutes
Ingredients:

- ¾ tsp soy sauce
- ¾ tsp rice wine

- ¾ tsp honey
- ¼ tsp five-spice
- 6 chicken wings
- ½ inch fresh ginger
- ½ inch ground mace
- 1 clove garlic, minced
- Sliced scallions for serving

Directions:

1. Prepare a water bath and place the Sous Vide in it. Set to 160 F.

2. In a bowl, combine the soy sauce, rice wine, honey, and five-spice. Place the chicken wings and garlic in a vacuum-sealable bag. Release air by the water displacement method, seal and submerge the bag in the water bath. Cook for 2 hours.

3. Once the timer has stopped, remove the wings and transfer to a baking tray. Bake in the oven for 5 minutes at 380 F. Serve on a platter and garnish with sliced scallions.

Crispy Chicken With Mushrooms

Servings: 4
Cooking Time: 1 Hour 15 Minutes

Ingredients:

- 4 boneless chicken breasts
- 1 cup panko bread crumbs
- 1 pound sliced Portobello mushrooms
- Small bunch of thyme
- 2 eggs
- Salt and black pepper to taste
- Canola oil to taste

Directions:

1. Prepare a water bath and place the Sous Vide in it. Set to 149 F.

2. Place the chicken in a vacuum-sealable bag. Season with salt and thyme. Release air by the water displacement method, seal and submerge in water bath. Cook for 60 minutes.

3. Meanwhile, heat a skillet over medium heat. Cook the mushrooms until the water has evaporated. Add in 3-4 sprigs of thyme. Season with salt and pepper. Once the timer has stopped, remove the bag.

4. Heat a frying pan with oil over medium heat. Mix the panko with salt and pepper. Layer the chicken in

panko mix. Fry for 1-2 minutes per side. Serve with mushrooms.

Turkey Breast With Crispy Skin

Cooking Time: 3 Hours 30 Minutes Cooking Temperature: 145°f

Ingredients:

- For Turkey Breast:
- 5-pound whole skin-on, bone-in turkey breast
- Kosher salt and freshly ground black pepper, to taste
- For Gravy:
- 1 tablespoon vegetable oil
- 2 celery ribs, roughly chopped
- 1 large carrot, peeled and roughly chopped
- 1 large onion, roughly chopped
- 4 cups low-sodium chicken broth
- 1 teaspoon soy sauce
- 2 bay leaves
- 3 tablespoons butter
- ¼ cup flour

Directions:

1. Attach the sous vide immersion circulator to a Cambro container or pot with water using an adjustable clamp and preheat water to 145°F.

2. Carefully remove turkey skin in a single piece and set aside. With a sharp boning knife, carefully remove meat from breastbone and set breastbone aside after chopping it into 1-inch chunks.

3. Season turkey breast generously with salt and black pepper. Place 1 breast half onto a smooth surface with the cut side facing up. Place second breast half with the cut side facing down and the fat end aligning with the skinny end of the first breast half. Gently roll up breast halves into an even cylinder and tie at 1-inch intervals with kitchen twine.

4. Place turkey roll in a cooking pouch. Seal pouch tightly after removing the excess air. Place pouch in sous vide bath and set the cooking time for 2½ hours.

5. Preheat oven to 400°F. Arrange a rack in the center position of the oven. Line a rimmed baking sheet with parchment paper.

6. For crispy skin: spread skin evenly onto prepared baking sheet. Season generously with salt

and black pepper. Arrange a second parchment paper over the turkey skin and carefully squeeze out any air bubbles with the side of your hand. Place another rimmed baking sheet on top of the parchment paper.

7. Roast for 30-45 minutes. Remove from oven and set aside to cool in room temperature.

8. For gravy: heat oil over high heat in a medium pan. Add chopped breastbone, celery, carrot, and onion and cook for 10 minutes, stirring occasionally.

9. Add broth, soy sauce, and bay leaves and bring to a boil. Reduce heat and simmer for 1 hour. Through a fine-mesh strainer, strain mixture. The broth should be a little over 4 cups. Discard solids from mixture and keep broth, setting aside.

10. in another medium pan, melt butter over medium heat. Add flour and cook for 3 minutes, stirring continuously. Slowly add broth, beating continuously, and bring to a boil. Reduce heat and simmer until mixture reduces to 3 cups. Season with salt and pepper.

11. Remove pouch from the sous vide bath and open carefully. Remove turkey roll from pouch and carefully remove kitchen twine.

12. Cut roll into ¼-½ inch slices. Break skin into serving-sized pieces. Place turkey slices onto a warmed serving platter with skin pieces arranged around and serve alongside gravy.

Coq Au Vin

Cooking Time: 12 Hours 30 Minutes Cooking Temperature: 151°f

Ingredients:

- 1 bottle red wine, reserving 1 glass
- 1/2 cup bacon, crumbled
- 3 large carrots, peeled and chopped
- 3 celery stalks, finely chopped
- 4 garlic cloves, pressed
- 4 bay leaves
- 7 tbsp unsalted butter, divided
- 10 shallots or small onions
- 1 chicken, jointed into 2 breasts on the bone with wings and 2 legs attached
- Sea salt and freshly ground black pepper, to taste
- A few thyme sprigs
- 2 tablespoons all-purpose flour
- Vegetable oil*
- 7 ounces button mushrooms
- Finely chopped fresh parsley, for garnishing

Directions:

1. Add wine, bacon, carrots, celery, garlic, and bay leaves to a pan and bring to a gentle boil. Cook for 25 minutes, stirring occasionally. Remove from heat and allow to cool completely.

2. Meanwhile in another pan, melt 1 tbsp butter and sauté onions for 4-5 minutes. Remove from heat and set aside.

3. Attach the sous vide immersion circulator to a Cambro container or pot with water using an adjustable clamp and preheat water to 151°F.

4. Season the jointed chickens evenly with salt and black pepper.

5. Divide chicken pieces, sautéed onions, and thyme sprigs between two cooking pouches. Seal pouches tightly after removing excess air. Place pouches in sous vide bath and set the cooking time for 12 hours.

6. Preheat the oven to 355°F.

7. Remove pouches from the sous vide bath and open carefully. Remove chicken pieces from pouches, reserving cooking liquid in a pan. Pat dry chicken pieces with paper towels.

8. Season chicken lightly with salt and pepper.

9. In a large frying pan, heat oil and 2 tablespoons butter. Add chicken, skin side down, and fry for 6-8 minutes on each side.

10. Move chicken pieces to a baking sheet, skin side up, and bake for 10 minutes.

11. While the chicken is baking, remove thyme sprigs from cooking liquid and bring liquid to a gentle boil, adding reserved wine.

12. In a bowl, combine flour and 2 tablespoons unsalted butter and mix well. Add flour mixture to pan with cooking liquid, stirring continuously. Stir in salt and black pepper and simmer until desired consistency is reached.

13. Move baked chicken pieces to a different pan on the stove. Add 2 tablespoons of butter and stir fry with mushrooms for 6-7 minutes or until browned on both sides.

14. Place chicken on a serving platter and top with sauce, followed by mushrooms. Garnish with parsley and serve.

Thai Green Curry Noodle Soup

Servings: 2
Cooking Time: 90 Minutes
Ingredients:
- 1 chicken breast, boneless and skinless
- Salt and pepper as needed
- 1 can /15 oz. coconut milk
- 2 tablespoons Thai Green Curry Paste
- 1¾ cups chicken stock
- 1 cup enoki mushrooms
- 5 kaffir lime leaves, torn in half
- 2 tablespoons fish sauce
- 1½ tablespoons palm sugar
- ½ cup Thai basil leaves, roughly chopped
- 2 oz cooked egg noodle nests
- 1 cup cilantro, roughly chopped
- 1 cup bean sprouts
- 2 tablespoons fried noodles
- 2 red Thai chilis, roughly chopped

Directions:
1. Prepare your water bath using your Sous Vide immersion circulator, and raise the temperature to 140-degrees Fahrenheit
2. Take the chicken and season it generously with salt and pepper and place it in a medium-sized, resealable bag with 1 tablespoon of coconut milk
3. Seal it using the immersion method and submerge. Cook for 90 minutes
4. After 35 minutes, place a medium-sized saucepan over a medium heat
5. Add the green curry paste and half the coconut milk
6. Bring the mix to a simmer and cook for 5-10 minutes until the coconut milk starts to show a beady texture
7. Add the chicken stock and the rest of the coconut milk and bring the mixture to a simmer once again, keep cooking for about 15 minutes
8. Add the kaffir lime leaves, enoki mushrooms, palm sugar and fish sauce

9. Lower the heat to medium-low and simmer for about 10 minutes
10. Remove from the heat and season with palm sugar and fish sauce, stir in the basil
11. Once the chicken is cooked fully, transfer it to a cooking board. Let it cool for few minutes and then cut into slices
12. Serve the chicken with the curry sauce and a topping of cooked egg noodles
13. Garnish the chicken with some bean sprouts, cilantro, Thai chilies and fried noodles. Serve!
Nutrition Info: Calories: 237 Carbohydrate: 21g Protein: 15g Fat: 11g Sugar: 5g Sodium: 567mg

Panko Crusted Chicken

Servings: 4
Cooking Time: 60 Minutes
Ingredients:
- 4 boneless chicken breasts
- 1 cup panko bread crumbs
- 1 lb. sliced mushrooms
- Small bunch of thyme
- 2 eggs
- Salt and pepper as needed
- Canola oil as needed

Directions:
1. Prepare your water bath using your Sous Vide immersion circulator, and increase the temperature to 150-degrees Fahrenheit
2. Season the chicken with salt, and thyme
3. Place the breast in a resealable bag and seal using the immersion method and cook for 60 minutes
4. Then, place a pan over medium heat, add the mushrooms and cook them until the water has evaporated
5. Add 3-4 sprigs of thyme and stir
6. Once cooked, remove the chicken from the bag and pat dry
7. Add the oil and heat it up over medium-high heat. Add the eggs into a container and dip the chicken in egg wash until well coated.
8. Add the panko bread crumbs in a shallow container and add some salt and pepper. Put the chicken to bread crumbs and coat until well covered.

9. Fry the chicken for 1-2 minutes per side and serve with the mushrooms
Nutrition Info: Per serving:Calories: 394 ;Carbohydrate: 71g ;Protein: 19g ;Fat: 5g ;Sugar: 5g ;Sodium: 59mg

Chicken & Leek Stew

Servings: 4
Cooking Time: 70 Minutes
Ingredients:
- 6 skinless chicken breasts
- Salt and black pepper to taste
- 3 tbsp butter
- 1 large leek, sliced crossways
- ½ cup panko
- 2 tbsp chopped parsley
- 1 oz Copoundy Jack cheese
- 1 tbsp olive oil

Directions:
1. Prepare a water bath and place the Sous Vide in it. Set to 146 F.
2. Place the chicken breasts in a vacuum-sealable bag. Season with salt and pepper. Release air by the water displacement method, seal and submerge in water bath. Cook for 45 minutes.
3. Meanwhile, heat a skillet over high heat with butter and cook the leeks. Season with salt and pepper. Mix well. Lower the heat and let cook for 10 minutes.
4. Heat a skillet over medium heat with butter and add the panko. Cook until toast. Transfer to a bowl and combine with cheddar cheese and chopped parsley. Once the timer has stopped, remove the breasts and pat dry. Heat a pan over high heat with olive oil and sear the chicken 1 minute per side. Serve over leeks and garnish with panko mix.

Chicken Salad

Cooking Time: 2 Hours Cooking Temperature: 150°f
Ingredients:
- 2 pounds chicken breast
- 2 tarragon sprigs
- 2 garlic cloves, smashed
- Zest and juice of 1 lemon

- Kosher salt and freshly ground black pepper, to taste
- ½ cup mayonnaise
- 1 tablespoon honey
- 1 celery stalk, minced
- 1 garlic clove, minced
- ½ Serrano Chile, stemmed, seeded, and minced
- 2 tablespoons fresh tarragon leaves, minced

Directions:
1. Attach the sous vide immersion circulator to a Cambro container or pot with water using an adjustable clamp and preheat water to 150°F.
2. Place chicken breasts, tarragon sprigs, smashed garlic cloves, lemon zest, salt, and pepper in a cooking pouch. Seal pouch tightly after removing the excess air. Place pouch in sous vide bath and set the cooking time for 2 hours.
3. Remove pouch from the sous vide bath and immediately plunge into a large bowl of ice water.
4. Once cooled completely, remove chicken breasts from pouch and transfer to a cutting board, discarding the tarragon sprigs, garlic, and lemon zest.
5. Roughly chop chicken and transfer place in a bowl. Add remaining ingredients and a little salt and black pepper and stir to combine. Serve immediately.

Singaporean Chicken Wings

Servings: 2
Cooking Time: 120 Minutes
Ingredients:
- ¾ teaspoon soy sauce
- ¾ teaspoon Chinese rice wine
- ¾ teaspoon honey
- ¼ teaspoon five-spice
- 2 whole chicken wings
- ½ inch fresh ginger
- 1 clove garlic, smashed
- Sliced scallions for serving

Directions:
1. Prepare your Sous Vide water bath using your immersion circulator, and raise the temperature to 160-degrees Fahrenheit
2. Add the soy sauce, rice wine, honey and five spice in a bowl and mix well

3. Place the chicken wings, garlic, ginger in a zip bag
4. Seal using the immersion method and cook for 120 minutes
5. Heat your broiler to high heat and line a broil-safe baking sheet with aluminum foil
6. Remove the wings and transfer to your broiling pan
7. Broil for 3-5 minutes
8. Then, arrange on a serving platter and sprinkle some sliced scallions over it
9. Serve!

Nutrition Info: Calories: 402 Carbohydrate: 11g Protein: 21g Fat: 18g Sugar: 6g Sodium: 340mg

Pheasant Breast

Servings: 2
Cooking Time: 45 Minutes
Ingredients:
- 2 pheasant breasts, bone in
- Kosher salt as needed
- Fresh ground black pepper to taste
- 2 tablespoons unsalted butter
- 3 sprigs of thyme
- 1 tablespoon extra-virgin olive oil

Directions:
1. Prepare your Sous Vide water bath, using your immersion circulator, and raise the temperature to 145-degrees Fahrenheit
2. Season the pheasant breast with pepper and salt and place them in a zip bag
3. Add the butter and thyme
4. Seal using the immersion method and cook for 45 minutes
5. Once done, remove the pheasant and pat dry
6. Discard the cooking liquid
7. Place a large, non-stick skillet over a medium heat and add the oil
8. Once the oil is heated, add the pheasant, skin side down, in the skillet
9. Sear for 2 minutes and serve!

Nutrition Info: Calories: 283 Carbohydrate: 3g Protein: 17g Fat: 21g Sugar: 71 Sodium: 145mg

Chicken Adobo

Cooking Time: 8 Hours Cooking Temperature: 160°f
Ingredients:
- 2 whole chicken legs, leg and thigh attached
- 4-5 garlic cloves, smashed
- ¼ cup cane vinegar or apple cider vinegar
- 2 tablespoons soy sauce
- 1 bay leaf
- ¼ teaspoon whole black peppercorns

Directions:
1. Attach the sous vide immersion circulator to a Cambro container or pot with water using an adjustable clamp and preheat water to 160°F.
2. Mix all ingredients together in a large cooking pouch. Seal pouch tightly after removing the excess air. Place pouch in sous vide bath and set the cooking time for 8 hours.
3. Preheat the oven broiler to high. Line a baking sheet with a piece of foil.
4. Remove pouch from the sous vide bath and open carefully. Remove the chicken legs from the pouch, reserving the cooking liquid in the pouch, and pat dry the chicken legs with paper towels.
5. Arrange chicken legs onto prepared baking sheet in a single layer. Broil for 3-6 minutes.
6. Add reserved cooking liquid to a small pan and bring to a gentle boil. Cook for 5 minutes.
7. Arrange chicken legs onto a serving platter and drizzle with sauce. Serve immediately.

Chicken Parmigiana

Cooking Time: 12 Hours Cooking Temperature: 141°f
Ingredients:
- For Chicken:
- 4 chicken breasts
- ½ teaspoon garlic powder
- Salt and freshly ground black pepper, to taste
- 4 fresh rosemary sprigs
- 4 fresh thyme sprigs
- For Coating:
- ¾ cup flour
- 2 teaspoons salt
- 1 teaspoon ground black pepper
- 2 eggs

42

- ¼ cup Parmesan cheese, grated
- ¾ cup dried Italian breadcrumbs
- 2 tablespoons fresh parsley, chopped
- For Cooking:
- Oil, as required
- For Topping:
- ½ cup fresh basil, chopped
- 1 cup fresh mozzarella cheese, shredded
- ¼ cup Parmesan cheese, grated

Directions:

1. Season chicken breasts with garlic powder, salt, and black pepper evenly.
2. Divide chicken breasts and herb sprigs into two cooking pouches. Seal pouches tightly after removing the excess air. Refrigerate pouches for up to 2 days.
3. Attach the sous vide immersion circulator to a Cambro container or pot with water using an adjustable clamp and preheat water to 141°F.
4. Place pouches in sous vide bath and set the cooking time for 2-12 hours.
5. Preheat the oven broiler.
6. Remove the pouches from the sous vide bath and open carefully. Remove the chicken breasts and pat dry chicken breasts completely with paper towels.
7. In a shallow dish, mix together flour, salt, and black pepper for coating. In a second shallow dish, beat eggs. In a third shallow dish, mix together Parmesan cheese, breadcrumbs, and parsley.
8. Coat chicken breasts evenly with flour mixture, then dip in egg mixture before coating with parmesan mixture.
9. In a deep skillet, heat ½-inch of oil to 350°F and sear chicken breasts until crust is golden brown then turn and repeat on other side.
10. Transfer chicken breasts to a sheet pan. Top each breast with the basil, Parmesan, and mozzarella cheese for topping. Broil until cheese is bubbly.
11. Serve immediately.

Herby Chicken With Butternut Squash Dish

Servings: 2
Cooking Time: 1 Hour 15 Minutes

Ingredients:

- 6 chicken tenderloin
- 4 cups butternut squash, cubed and roasted
- 4 cups rocket lettuce
- 4 tbsp sliced almonds
- Juice of 1 lemon
- 2 tbsp olive oil
- 4 tbsp red onion, chopped
- 1 tbsp paprika
- 1 tbsp turmeric
- 1 tbsp cumin
- Salt to taste

Directions:

1. Prepare a water bath and place the Sous Vide in it. Set to 138 F.
2. Place the chicken and all seasonings in a vacuum-sealable bag. Release air by the water displacement method, seal and submerge in water bath. Cook for 60 minutes.
3. Once the timer has stopped, remove the bag and transfer the chicken to a hot skillet. Sear for 1 minute per side. In a bowl, combine the remaining ingredients. Serve the chicken with the salad.

Stuffed Cornish Hen

Servings: 5
Cooking Time: 4 Hours

Ingredients:

- 2 whole Cornish game hens
- 4 tablespoons unsalted butter plus 1 tablespoon extra, melted
- 2 cups shitake mushrooms, thinly sliced
- 1 cup leeks, finely diced
- ¼ cup walnuts, coarsely chopped
- 1 tablespoon fresh thyme, minced
- 1 cup cooking wild rice
- ¼ cup dried cranberries
- 1 tablespoon honey

Directions:

1. Prepare your water bath using your Sous Vide immersion circulator, and raise the temperature to 150-degrees Fahrenheit

2. Take a large sized skillet and place it over medium heat

3. Once the skillet is hot, add 3 tablespoons of butter and allow the butter to melt

4. Add the mushrooms, thyme, leek and walnuts and cook for 5-10 minutes

5. Stir in the rice, cranberries and remove from the heat, allow to cool for 10 minutes

6. Divide the stuffing between the hen cavities

7. Truss the legs together tightly and put the hens in a zip bag

8. Seal using the immersion method and cook for 4 hours

9. Remove the hens and pat dry

10. Set your broiler to high heat

11. Add the honey and the extra tablespoon of melted butter in a small bowl

12. Brush the mixture over the hens

13. Broil for 2 minutes and then serve

Nutrition Info: Calories: 1196 Carbohydrate: 70g Protein: 69g Fat: 72g Sugar: 11g Sodium: 523mg

Oregano Chicken Meatballs

Servings: 4
Cooking Time: 2 Hours 20 Minutes
Ingredients:

- 1 pound ground chicken
- 1 tbsp olive oil
- 2 garlic cloves, minced
- 1 tsp fresh oregano, minced
- Salt to taste
- 1 tbsp cumin
- ½ tsp grated lemon zest
- ½ tsp black pepper
- ¼ cup panko breadcrumbs
- Lemon wedges

Directions:

1. Prepare a water bath and place Sous Vide in it. Set to 146 F. Combine in a bowl ground chicken, garlic, olive oil, oregano, lemon zest, cumin, salt, and pepper. Using your hands make at least 14 meatballs. Place the meatballs in a vacuum-sealable bag. Release air by the water displacement method, seal

and submerge the bag in the water bath. Cook for 2 hours.

2. Once the timer has stopped, remove the bag and transfer the meatballs to a baking sheet, lined with foil. Heat a skillet over medium heat and sear the meatballs for 7 minutes. Top with lemon wedges.

Simple Spicy Chicken Thighs

Servings: 6
Cooking Time: 2 Hours 55 Minutes
Ingredients:

- 1 lb chicken thighs, bone-in
- 3 tbsp butter
- 1 tbsp cayenne pepper
- Salt to taste

Directions:

1. Make a water bath, place Sous Vide in it, and set to 165 F. Season the chicken with pepper and salt. Place chicken with one tablespoon of butter in a vacuum-sealable bag. Release air by the water displacement method, seal and submerge the bag in the water bath. Set the timer for 2 hours 30 minutes.

2. Once the timer has stopped, remove the bag and unseal it. Preheat a grill and melt the remaining butter in a microwave. Grease the grill grate with some of the butter and brush the chicken with the remaining butter. Sear until dark brown color is achieved. Serve as a snack.

Fried Chicken

Servings: 4
Cooking Time: 1 Hour
Ingredients:

- 8 pieces chicken, legs or thighs
- Salt and pepper as needed
- Lemon wedges for serving
- For Wet Mix
- 2 cups soy milk
- 1 tablespoon lemon juice
- For Dry Mix
- 1 cup plain, high protein flour
- 1 cup rice flour

- ½ cup cornstarch
- 2 tablespoons paprika
- 2 tablespoons salt
- 2 tablespoons ground black pepper

Directions:

1. Prepare your sous vide water bath to a temperature of 154-degrees Fahrenheit, using your immersion circulator
2. Season your chicken pieces well with pepper and salt and seal them in a resealable bag using the water immersion method
3. Cook them in the water bath for 1 hour
4. Remove the chicken and place it to one side. Allow it to sit for 15-20 minutes
5. Take a pan and place it on the stove, pour in some oil and pre-heat to a temperature of 400-425-degrees Fahrenheit
6. Take a large-sized bowl and add the soy milk and lemon juice, whisk them well
7. Use another bowl to mix the protein flour, rice flour, cornstarch, paprika, salt and ground black pepper
8. Gently dip the cooked chicken in the dry mix, then dip into the wet mixture
9. Repeat 2-3 times then place the prepared chickens on a wire rack
10. Keep repeating until all the chicken has been used
11. Fry the chicken in small batches for about 3-4 minutes for each batch
12. Once done, allow the chicken to cool on the wire rack for 10-15 minutes
13. Serve with some lemon wedges and sauce!

Nutrition Info: Calories: 251 Carbohydrate: 10g Protein: 28g Fat: 11g Sugar: 4g Sodium: 458mg Special Tips It is wise to rub the turkey legs with olive oil before searing them. This will allow them to take on a much crispier texture and help avoid burning.

Rosemary Chicken Stew

Servings: 2
Cooking Time: 4 Hours 15 Minutes
Ingredients:

- 2 chicken thighs
- 6 garlic cloves, crushed
- ¼ tsp whole black pepper
- 2 bay leaves
- ¼ cup dark soy sauce
- ¼ cup white vinegar
- 1 tbsp rosemary

Directions:

1. Prepare a water bath and place the Sous Vide in it. Set to 165 F. Combine the chicken thighs with all the ingredients. Place in a vacuum-sealable bag. Release air by the water displacement method, seal and submerge in water bath. Cook for 4 hours.
2. Once the timer has stopped, remove the chicken, discard bay leaves and reserve the cooking juices. Heat canola oil in a skillet over medium heat and sear the chicken. Add in cooking juices and cook until you have reached the desired consistency. Filter the sauce and top the chicken.

Savory Lettuce Wraps With Ginger-chili Chicken

Servings: 5
Cooking Time: 1 Hour 45 Minutes
Ingredients:

- ½ cup hoisin sauce
- ½ cup sweet chili sauce
- 3 tbsp soy sauce
- 2 tbsp grated ginger
- 2 tbsp ground ginger
- 1 tbsp brown sugar
- 2 garlic cloves, minced
- Juice of 1 lime
- 4 chicken breasts, cubed
- Salt and black pepper to taste
- 12 lettuce leaves, rinsed
- ⅛ cup poppy seeds
- 4 chives

Directions:

1. Prepare a water bath and place Sous Vide in it. Set to 141 F. Combine chili sauce, ginger, soy sauce, brown sugar, garlic, and half of lime juice. Heat a

saucepan over medium heat and pour in the mixture. Cook for 5 minutes. Set aside.

2. Season the breasts with salt and pepper. Place them in an even layer in a vacuum-sealable bag with the chili sauce mixture. Release air by the water displacement method, seal and submerge the bag in the water bath. Cook for 1 hour and 30 minutes.

3. Once the timer has stopped, remove the chicken and pat dry with kitchen towel. Discard cooking juices. Combine the hoisin sauce with the chicken cubes and mix well. Make piles of 6 lettuce leaves.

4. Share chicken among lettuce leaves and top with the poppy seeds and chives before wrapping.

Prosciutto Wrapped Chicken

Cooking Time: 1 Hour 5 Minutes Cooking Temperature: 145°f

Ingredients:

*   2 (6-ounce) boneless, skinless chicken breasts, sliced in half lengthwise
*   Kosher salt and freshly ground black pepper, to taste
*   2 thin prosciutto slices
*   1 tablespoon extra-virgin olive oil

Directions:

1. Attach the sous vide immersion circulator to a Cambro container or pot with water using an adjustable clamp and preheat water to 145°F.

2. Season chicken breasts evenly with salt and black pepper.

3. Arrange a piece of plastic wrap onto a cutting board. Place one prosciutto slice in the center of the plastic wrap. Arrange two of the strips of chicken in the center of prosciutto, side-by-side to form an even rectangle. Roll prosciutto around the chicken so that it creates a uniform cylinder. Wrap the cylinder tightly in the plastic wrap and tie off the ends with butcher's twine. Repeat with remaining prosciutto and chicken.

4. Place the chicken cylinders in a large cooking pouch. Seal pouch tightly after removing the excess air. Place the pouch in the sous vide bath and set the cooking time for 1 hour.

5. Remove pouch from the sous vide bath and open carefully. Remove the chicken cylinders from the pouch and take off the plastic wrap, patting dry the chicken cylinders. Season each cylinder with salt and black pepper.

6. In a large, non-stick skillet, heat olive oil over medium-high heat and sear chicken cylinders for 5 minutes or until golden brown.

7. Remove from heat and allow to cool for 10 minutes. Cut into desired slices and serve.

Chicken With Vegetables

Servings: 2
Cooking Time: 2 Hours 15 Minutes
Ingredients:

*   1 pound chicken breasts, boneless and skinless
*   1 cup red bell pepper, sliced
*   1 cup green bell pepper, sliced
*   1 cup zucchini, sliced
*   ½ cup onion, finely chopped
*   1 cup cauliflower florets
*   ½ cup freshly squeezed lemon juice
*   ½ cup chicken stock
*   ½ tsp ground ginger
*   1 tsp pink Himalayan salt

Directions:

1. In a bowl, combine lemon juice with chicken stock, ginger, and salt. Stir well and add sliced vegetables. Set aside. Rinse well the chicken breast under cold running water. Using a sharp paring knife, cut the meat into bite-sized pieces.

2. Combine with other ingredients and stir well. Transfer to a large vacuum-sealable bag and seal. Cook en Sous Vide for 2 hours at 167 F. Serve immediately.

Artichoke Stuffed Chicken

Servings: 6
Cooking Time: 3hours 15 Minutes
Ingredients:

*   2 pounds chicken breast fillets, butterfly cut
*   ½ cup chopped baby spinach

- 8 garlic cloves, crushed
- 10 artichoke hearts
- Salt and white pepper to taste
- 4 tbsp olive oil

Directions:

1. Combine artichoke, pepper, and garlic in a food processor. Blend until completely smooth. Pulse again and gradually add oil until well incorporated.

2. Stuff each breast with equal amounts of artichoke mixture and chopped baby spinach. Fold the breast fillet back together and secure the edge with a wooden skewer. Season with salt and white pepper and transfer to a separate vacuum-sealable bags. Seal the bags and cook en Sous Vide for 3 hours at 149 F.

Rare Duck Breast

Servings: 2
Cooking Time: 120 Minutes
Ingredients:

- 2 duck breasts
- ¼ cup olive oil
- 4 sprigs thyme
- Salt and pepper as needed

Directions:

1. Prepare your Sous Vide water bath using your immersion circulator and raise the temperature to 135-degrees Fahrenheit

2. Transfer the duck breast to a hot pan and sear them for 1-2 minutes per side

3. Place in a zip bag with the olive oil and thyme

4. Cook for 2 hours

5. Sear them again for 1-2 minutes in a hot pan

6. Allow them to rest and slice

7. Sprinkle with salt and pepper and serve

Nutrition Info: Per serving:Calories: 434 ;Carbohydrate: 8g ;Protein: 47g ;Fat: 24g ;Sugar: 1g ;Sodium: 645mg

Chicken Thighs With Garlic Mustard Sauce

Cooking Time: 4 Hours 10 Minutes Cooking Temperature: 165°f

Ingredients:

- 1½ pound skin-on chicken thighs
- Salt and freshly ground black pepper, to taste
- 2 tablespoons canola oil
- 1 tablespoon butter
- 1 teaspoon champagne or white wine vinegar
- 1 large garlic clove, mashed into a paste
- 1 teaspoon whole-grain Dijon mustard

Directions:

1. Attach the sous vide immersion circulator to a Cambro container or pot with water using an adjustable clamp and preheat water to 165°F.

2. Season chicken generously with salt and pepper.

3. Place chicken in a cooking pouch and seal pouch tightly after removing the excess air. Place pouch in sous vide bath and set the cooking time for 1-4 hours.

4. Remove pouch from the sous vide bath and open carefully. Transfer chicken to a plate, reserving the cooking liquid from the pouch.

5. In a large non-stick skillet, heat oil over high heat. Place chicken skin side down and cook for 2-3 minutes. Transfer chicken to a plate and set aside.

6. Wipe out skillet with paper towels then melt butter over low heat. Add reserved cooking liquid and remaining ingredients and simmer until sauce becomes thick.

7. Place sauce over chicken and serve.

Classic Chicken Cordon Bleu

Servings: 4
Cooking Time: 1 Hour 50 Minutes + Cooling Time
Ingredients:

- ½ cup butter
- 4 boneless, skinless chicken breasts
- Salt and black pepper to taste
- 1 tsp cayenne pepper
- 4 garlic cloves, minced
- 8 slices ham
- 8 slices Emmental cheese

Directions:

1. Prepare a water bath and place the Sous Vide in it. Set to 141 F. Season the chicken with salt and

pepper. Cover with plastic wrap and rolled. Set aside and allow to chill.

2.   Heat a saucepan over medium heat and add some black pepper, cayenne pepper, 1/4 cup of butter, and garlic. Cook until the butter melts. Transfer to a bowl.

3.   Rub the chicken on one side with the butter mixture. Then place 2 slices of ham and 2 slices of cheese and cover it. Roll each breast with plastic wrap and transfer to the fridge for 2-3 hours or in the freezer for 20-30 minutes.

4.   Place the breast in two vacuum-sealable bags. Release air by the water displacement method, seal and submerge the bags in the water bath. Cook for 1 hour and 30 minutes.

5.   Once the timer has stopped, remove the breasts and take off the plastic. Heat the remaining butter in a skillet over medium heat and sear the chicken for 1-2 minutes per side.

Shredded Chicken Patties

Servings: 5
Cooking Time: 3 Hours 15 Minutes
Ingredients:
- ½ lb chicken breast, skinless and boneless
- ½ cup macadamia nuts, grounded
- ⅓ cup olive oil mayonnaise
- 3 green onions, finely chopped
- 2 tbsp lemon juice
- Salt and black pepper to taste
- 3 tbsp olive oil

Directions:

1.   Make a water bath, place Sous Vide in it, and set to 165 F. Put chicken in a vacuum-sealable bag, release air by the water displacement method and seal it. Put the bag in the water bath and set the timer for 3 hours. Once the timer has stopped, remove and unseal the bag.

2.   Shred the chicken and add it to a bowl along with all the remaining ingredients except olive oil. Mix evenly and and make patties. Heat olive oil in a skillet over medium heat. Add patties and fry to golden brown on both sides.

Chicken Roulade

Servings: 2
Cooking Time: 90 Minutes
Ingredients:
- 1 x 8 oz chicken breast
- ¼ cup goat cheese
- ¼ cup julienned roasted red pepper
- ½ cup loosely packed arugula
- 6 slices prosciutto
- Salt and pepper as needed
- 1 tablespoon oil for searing
- Tools Required: Plastic wrap, wine/vinegar bottle

Directions:

1.   Prepare your water bath, using your Sous Vide immersion circulator, and raise the temperature to 155-degrees Fahrenheit

2.   Drain the chicken breast if needed, and place it between plastic wrap. Pound it using a mallet or the side of wine bottle, until it gets ¼ inch thick

3.   Cut in half and season both sides with pepper and salt

4.   Spread 2 tablespoons of goat cheese on top and top each half with roasted red peppers

5.   Top with half the arugula

6.   Roll both breasts like sushi

7.   Place 3 layers of prosciutto on your work surface /overlapping each other

8.   Put the rolled chicken at the base of the prosciutto and roll it all up to enclose the roulade

9.   Place in a zip bag and seal using the immersion method and cook for 90 minutes

10.   Take out of the bag and sear

11.   Slice and then serve

Nutrition Info: Calories: 513 Carbohydrate: 6g Protein: 47g Fat: 32g Sugar: 2g Sodium: 527mg

Green Chicken Salad With Almonds

Servings: 2
Cooking Time: 95 Minutes
Ingredients:

- 2 chicken breasts, skinless
- Salt and black pepper to taste
- 1 cup almonds
- 1 tbsp olive oil
- 2 tbsp sugar
- 4 red chilis, thinly sliced
- 1 garlic clove, peeled
- 3 tbsp fish sauce
- 2 tsp freshly squeezed lime juice
- 1 cup cilantro, chopped
- 1 scallion, thinly sliced
- 1 stalk lemongrass, white part only, sliced
- 1 piece 2-inch ginger, julienned

Directions:

1. Prepare a water bath and place the Sous Vide in it. Set to 138 F. Place the chicken seasoned with salt and pepper in a vacuum-sealable bag. Release air by the water displacement method, seal and submerge the bag in the water bath. Cook for 75 minutes.
2. After 60 minutes, heat olive oil in a saucepan to 350 F. Toast the almonds for 1 minute until dry. Batter the sugar, garlic and chili. Pour in fish sauce and lime juice.
3. Once ready, remove the bag and let cool. Cut the chicken in bites and place in a bowl. Pour the dressing and mix well. Add the cilantro, ginger, lemongrass and fried almonds. Garnish with chili and serve.

Aji Amarillo Chicken Wings

Cooking Time: 4 Hours 15 Minutes Cooking Temperature: 160°f

Ingredients:

- For Sauce:
- 1 teaspoon olive oil
- ½ white onion, chopped
- 3 Aji Amarillo peppers, seeded and roughly chopped
- 2 garlic cloves, chopped
- 2 tablespoons white vinegar
- Salt and freshly ground black pepper, to taste
- For Wings:
- 40 split chicken wings

- Salt and freshly ground black pepper, to taste

Directions:

1. Attach the sous vide immersion circulator to a Cambro container or pot with water using an adjustable clamp and preheat water to 160°F.
2. For sauce: in a pan, heat oil over medium heat and sauté onion, peppers, and garlic until onion is translucent and peppers softened.
3. Transfer mixture to a blender, add vinegar, salt, and black pepper, and pulse until smooth. Reserve 1 tablespoon of sauce in a bowl.
4. Season chicken wings lightly with salt and black pepper.
5. Place chicken wings and all but the 1 tablespoon of reserved sauce in a cooking pouch. Seal pouch tightly after removing the excess air. Place pouch in sous vide bath and set the cooking time for 4 hours.
6. Preheat the oven broiler to high. Line a baking sheet with parchment paper.
7. Remove pouch from the sous vide bath and open carefully, removing chicken wings from pouch.
8. Arrange chicken wings onto the prepared baking sheet in a single layer. Broil for 10-15 minutes, flipping once halfway through the cooking time.
9. Remove from oven and transfer into bowl of reserved sauce. Toss to coat well and serve immediately.

Mustard & Garlic Chicken

Servings: 5
Cooking Time: 60 Minutes

Ingredients:

- 17 ounces chicken breasts
- 1 tbsp Dijon mustard
- 2 tbsp mustard powder
- 2 tsp tomato sauce
- 3 tbsp butter
- 1 tsp salt
- 3 tsp minced garlic
- ¼ cup soy sauce

Directions:

1. Prepare a water bath and place the Sous Vide in it. Set to 150 F. Place all the ingredients in a vacuum-

sealable bag and shake to combine. Release air by the water displacement method, seal and submerge the bag in water bath.Set the timer for 50 minutes. Once the timer has stopped, remove the chicken and slice. Serve warm.

Tandoori Chicken

Cooking Time: 1 Hour 40 Minutes Cooking Temperature: 140°f

Ingredients:
- 7 tablespoons tandoori paste, divided
- 3 teaspoons ghee
- 5 boneless, skinless chicken thighs, sliced into bite-sized pieces
- 2 tablespoons plain yogurt
- 1 teaspoon cumin seeds
- Vegetable oil, as required
- Metal skewers or soaked wooden skewers, for grilling
- Your favorite dipping sauce, for serving

Directions:
1. Attach the sous vide immersion circulator to a Cambro container or pot with water using an adjustable clamp and preheat water to 140°F.
2. In a small bowl, mix 5 tablespoons of tandoori paste and ghee. Coat chicken thighs evenly with ghee mixture.
3. Place chicken thighs in a cooking pouch. Seal pouch tightly after removing the excess air. Place pouch in sous vide bath and set the cooking time for 1½ hours.
4. For sauce: in a large bowl, add remaining 2 tablespoons tandoori paste, yogurt, and cumin seeds and mix until well combined. Cover the bowl and set aside.
5. Grease a grill pan with oil and heat over high heat.
6. Remove pouch from the sous vide bath and open carefully. Remove chicken thighs from pouch into the bowl with the sauce and toss to coat.
7. Thread the chicken onto skewers and sear on grill pan for 30 seconds on each side.

8. Remove chicken from skewers and divide onto serving plates. Serve with your favorite dipping sauce.

Delicious Chicken Wings With Buffalo Sauce

Servings: 3
Cooking Time: 3 Hours
Ingredients:
- 3 pounds capon chicken wings
- 2½ cups buffalo sauce
- 1 bunch fresh parsley

Directions:
1. Prepare a water bath and place the Sous Vide in it. Set to 148 F.
2. Combine the capon wings with salt and pepper. Place it in a vacuum-sealable bag with 2 cups of buffalo sauce. Release air by the water displacement method, seal and submerge the bag in the water bath. Cook for 2 hours. Heat the oven to broil.
3. Once the timer has stopped, remove the wings and transfer into a bowl. Pour the remaining buffalo sauce and mix well. Transfer the wings to a baking tray with aluminium foil and cover with the remaining sauce. Bake for 10 minutes, turning at least once. Garnish with parsley.

Chicken Breasts With Harissa Sauce

Servings: 4
Cooking Time: 65 Minutes
Ingredients:
- 1 pound chicken breasts, cubed
- 1 stalk of fresh lemongrass, chopped
- 2 tbsp fish sauce
- 2 tbsp coconut sugar
- Salt to taste
- 1 tbsp harissa sauce

Directions:
1. Prepare a water bath and place the Sous Vide in it. Set to 149 F. In a blender, pulse lemongrass, fish sauce, sugar, and salt. Marinade the chicken with the sauce and make brochettes. Place it in a vacuum-

sealable bag. Release air by the water displacement method, seal and submerge the bag in the water bath. Cook for 45 minutes.

2.   Once the timer has stopped, remove the bag and transfer to a cold water bath. Remove the chicken and whisk with harissa sauce. Heat a skillet over medium heat and sear the chicken. Serve.

Chicken Breast Meal

Servings: 2

Cooking Time: 60 Minutes

Ingredients:

- 1-piece boneless chicken breast
- Salt and pepper as needed
- Garlic powder as needed

Directions:

1.   Prepare your water bath using your Sous Vide immersion circulator, and increase the temperature to 150-degrees Fahrenheit

2.   Carefully drain the chicken breast and pat dry using a kitchen towel

3.   Season the breast with garlic powder, pepper and salt

4.   Place in a resealable bag and seal using the immersion method

5.   Submerge and cook for 1 hour

6.   Serve!

Nutrition Info: Per serving:Calories: 150 ;Carbohydrate: 0g ;Protein: 18g ;Fat: 8g ;Sugar: 0g ;Sodium: 257mg

BEEF,PORK & LAMB RECIPES

Brined Bbq Ribs

Cooking Time: 24 Hours Cooking Temperature: 155°f

Ingredients:

- For Brine:
- 3-4 pounds Pork spare ribs
- 6 cups water
- 1/2 cup brown sugar
- 1/2 cup salt
- For Spice Rub:
- 3 teaspoons dried basil
- 2 teaspoons brown sugar
- 2 teaspoons white sugar
- 3 teaspoons garlic powder
- 3 teaspoons paprika
- 3 teaspoons ancho chiles
- 2 teaspoons salt
- 1 teaspoon cumin seeds
- Freshly ground black pepper, to taste
- For Serving:
- BBQ sauce (of your choice)

Directions:

1. Cut each rib into 3-4 rib portions.
2. For brine: add water, sugar, and salt to a large bowl and stir until sugar and salt dissolve completely. Add pork ribs, cover, and refrigerate for 24 hours.
3. Attach the sous vide immersion circulator to a Cambro container or pot with water using an adjustable clamp and preheat water to 155°F.
4. For spice rub: mix all spice rub ingredients together in a bowl.
5. Drain ribs and rinse under cold running water then pat dry ribs with paper towels. Season all ribs generously with spice rub.
6. Place each rib portion into a cooking pouch. Seal pouches tightly after removing the excess air. Place pouches in sous vide bath and set the cooking time for 24 hours. During cooking, cover the sous vide bath with plastic wrap to minimize water evaporation. Add water intermittently to keep the water level up.
7. Remove pouches from the sous vide bath and open carefully. Remove rib portions from pouches and pat dry ribs completely with paper towels.
8. Preheat grill to high heat.
9. Grill each rib portion until browned on both sides.
10. Serve immediately with your favorite BBQ sauce.

Honey Mustard Pork

Servings: 2
Cooking Time: 3 Hours

Ingredients:

- 3 tablespoons extra-virgin olive oil
- 1 tablespoon + 2 teaspoons whole grain mustard
- 1 tablespoon + 1 teaspoon honey
- Salt and ground black pepper, as needed
- 2 pieces' bone-in pork loin chops
- 1 tablespoon freshly squeezed lemon juice
- 2 teaspoons red wine vinegar
- 2 tablespoons rice bran oil
- 2 cups mixed baby lettuce
- 2 tablespoons thinly sliced sundried tomatoes
- 2 teaspoons pine nuts, toasted

Directions:

1. Prepare the Sous Vide water bath using the immersion circulator and raise the temperature to 140-degrees Fahrenheit.
2. Take a small bowl and mix in 1 tablespoon olive oil, 1 tablespoon mustard, 1 tablespoon honey, and season with salt and pepper
3. Transfer to a resealable zip bag alongside the pork chop and toss well to coat it.
4. Seal using the immersion method and cook for 3 hours.
5. To prepare the dressing, add the lemon juice, vinegar, 2 tablespoons of olive oil, 2 teaspoons of mustard and the remaining honey in a bowl. Season with salt and pepper.
6. Remove the bag and remove the pork chop, discard the liquid.
7. Take a large skillet over high heat and add bran oil, heat it up and wait until it starts to smoke. Add the pork chops and sear for 30 seconds per side.
8. Rest for 5 minutes.
9. Take a medium bowl and add the lettuce, sun-dried tomatoes and pine nuts, toss well with 3 quarter of the dressing.

10. Take the pork chops and transfer them to your serving plate and top with the salad and dressing.
11. Serve!

Nutrition Info: Per serving:Calories: 357 ;Carbohydrate: 22g ;Protein: 47g ;Fat: 8g ;Sugar: 22g ;Sodium: 162mg

Flavorful Pork With Mustard & Molasses Glaze

Servings: 6
Cooking Time: 4 Hours 15 Minutes
Ingredients:
- 2 pounds pork loin roast
- 1 bay leaf
- 3 oz molasses
- ½ oz soy sauce
- ½ oz honey
- Juice of 2 lemons
- 2 strips lemon peel
- 4 chopped scallions
- ½ tsp garlic powder
- ¼ tsp Dijon mustard
- ¼ tsp ground allspice
- 1 oz crushed corn chips

Directions:
1. Prepare a water bath and place the Sous Vide in it. Set to 142 F.
2. Place the pork loin and bay leaf in a vacuum-sealable bag. Add in molasses, soy sauce, lemon peel, honey, scallions, garlic powder, mustard, and allspice and shake well. Release air by the water displacement method, seal and submerge the bag in the water bath. Cook for 4 hours.
3. Once the timer has stopped, remove the bag. Pour the remaining mixture into a saucepan and boil until reduced. Serve the pork with the sauce and top with crushed corn chips. Garnish with green onion.

Savory Pork Chops With Mushrooms

Servings: 2
Cooking Time: 65 Minutes
Ingredients:
- 2 thick-cut bone-in pork chops
- Salt and black pepper to taste

- 2 tbsp butter, cold
- 4 oz mixed wild mushrooms
- ¼ cup sherry
- ½ cup beef stock
- 1 tsp sage
- 1 tbsp steak marinade
- Chopped garlic for garnish

Directions:
1. Prepare a water bath and place the Sous Vide in it. Set to 138 F.
2. Combine the pork with salt and pepper and place in a vacuum-sealable bag. Release air by the water displacement method, seal and submerge the bag in the water bath. Cook for 45 minutes.
3. Once the timer has stopped, remove the pork and dry it. Discard cooking juices. Heat 1 tbsp of butter in a skillet over medium heat and sear the pork for 1 minute each side. Transfer to a plate and set aside.
4. In the same hot skillet, cook the mushrooms for 2-3 minutes. Stir in sherry, stock, sage and steak marinade until the sauce thickens. Add in remaining butter and season with salt and pepper; stir well. Top the pork with the sauce and garnish with garlic chives to serve.

Venison Loin With Hazelnut Coffee Maple Butter

Cooking Time: 2 Hours Cooking Temperature: 140°f
Ingredients:
- For Venison Loin:
- 1-2 pound venison loin
- 3 garlic cloves, thinly sliced
- kosher salt, to taste
- freshly ground black pepper, to taste
- 1 tablespoon cumin seeds
- butter or fat of choice, as required
- For Hazelnut Coffee Maple Butter:
- ¼ cup unsalted butter, chopped
- 1½ tablespoons cool hazelnut coffee
- 1 tablespoon maple syrup

Directions:
1. Attach the sous vide immersion circulator using an adjustable clamp to a Cambro container or pot filled with water and preheat to 140°F.

2. Coat venison loin generously with cumin seeds, salt and black pepper. Place garlic slices over loin.

3. Into a cooking pouch, add venison loin. Seal pouch tightly after squeezing out the excess air. Place pouch in sous vide bath and set the cooking time for 2 hours.

4. Into a small food processor, add butter, hazelnut coffee and maple syrup, and pulse until well-combined.

5. Transfer butter mixture onto a wax paper and roll into a cylinder. Refrigerate for at least 1 hour.

6. Remove from the refrigerator and keep aside to come to room temperature. Cut into slices.

7. Remove pouch from sous vide bath and carefully open it. Remove venison loin from pouch. With paper towels, pat venison loin completely dry.

8. In a cast iron skillet, melt butter over medium-high heat, and sear venison loin for 30 seconds per side or until golden brown.

9. Season with salt and pepper, and transfer onto a cutting board.

10. Cut into medallions. Top with coffee butter and serve.

Pork Cheek Ragout

Servings: 8
Cooking Time: 10 Hours
Ingredients:
- 2 lbs. skinless pork cheeks
- 2 finely diced carrots
- ½ white onion, finely diced
- 1 cup canned tomato sauce
- 1 cup canned diced tomatoes
- 3 sprigs oregano
- 3 garlic cloves, crushed
- 1 teaspoon granulated sugar
- 2 pieces' bay leaves
- Kosher salt and black pepper, as needed
- Cooked pasta and fresh parsley for serving

Directions:
1. Prepare the Sous Vide water bath using your immersion circulator and raise the temperature to 180-degrees Fahrenheit.

2. Add the pork cheeks, carrots, onion, tomato sauce, diced tomatoes, garlic, oregano, sugar, bay leaves, 1 teaspoon of pepper, 1 tablespoon of salt to a heavy-duty re-sealable zip bag.

3. Seal using the immersion method. Cook for 10 hours.

4. Once done, remove the bag and then the pork, make sure to reserve the cooking liquid.

5. Shred using 2 forks into 1-inch pieces, transfer to large bowl and set it to the side.

6. Remove and discard the oregano from the cooking liquid, pour the contents to a food processor and pulse until the ingredients are uniformly chopped.

7. Take the sauce and season it well with pepper and salt, pour it over the pork toss to combine.

8. Toss the pasta with the mixture and serve with parsley!

Nutrition Info: Per serving:Calories: 428 ;Carbohydrate: 40g ;Protein: 26g ;Fat: 20g ;Sugar: 24g ;Sodium: 144mg

Bacon Strips & Eggs

Servings: 2
Cooking Time: 60 Minutes
Ingredients:
- 4 egg yolks
- 2 slices British-style bacon rashers cut up into ½ inch by 3-inch slices
- 4 slices crisp toasted bread

Directions:
1. Prepare the Sous Vide water bath using your immersion circulator and raise the temperature to 143-degrees Fahrenheit.

2. Gently place each of your egg yolks in the resealable zipper bag and seal it using the immersion method.

3. Submerge it underwater and cook for about 1 hour.

4. In the meantime, fry your bacon slices until they are crisp.

5. Drain them on a kitchen towel.

6. Once the eggs are cooked, serve by carefully removing the yolks from the zip bag and placing it on top of the toast.

7. Top with the slices of bacon and serve!

Nutrition Info: Per serving:Calories: 385 ;Carbohydrate: 49g ;Protein: 16g ;Fat: 16g ;Sugar: 4g ;Sodium: 514mg

Char Sui (chinese Pork)

Cooking Time: 15 Hours 5 Minutes Cooking Temperature: 155°f

Ingredients:

- For Pork Shoulder:
- 2 tablespoons caster sugar
- 2 cubes Chinese red fermented bean curd
- 2 teaspoons Chinese rose wine
- 1 tablespoon mild honey
- 1 tablespoon oyster sauce
- 1 tablespoon hoisin sauce
- 1 teaspoon soy sauce
- 1 teaspoon Chinese five spice powder
- ¼ teaspoon ground white pepper
- large pork shoulder
- For Glaze:
- 1 tablespoon honey

Directions:

1.   Attach the sous vide immersion circulator to a Cambro container or pot with water using an adjustable clamp and preheat water to 155°F.

2.   For pork shoulder: in a large bowl, add all ingredients for pork shoulder except the meat and mix until well combined. Add pork shoulder and coat generously with marinade.

3.   Place the pork shoulder in a cooking pouch with the marinade. Seal pouch tightly after removing the excess air. Place pouch in sous vide bath and set the cooking time for 15 hours. Cover the sous vide bath with plastic wrap to minimize water evaporation. Add water intermittently to keep the water level up.

4.   Preheat the oven broiler to high.

5.   Remove pouch from the sous vide bath and open carefully. Remove pork shoulder from pouch, reserving 1-2 tablespoons of the cooking liquid.

6.   For glaze: in a small bowl, mix together reserved cooking liquid and honey. Coat pork shoulder with glaze mixture.

7.   Transfer pork shoulder onto a roasting pan. Broil until charred on both sides.

8.   Remove from oven. Cut into slices of the desired size and serve.

Santa Maria Tri-tip

Cooking Time: 2 Hours Cooking Temperature: 135°f

Ingredients:

- 1½ tablespoons garlic salt with dried parsley
- 1 tablespoon freshly ground black pepper
- 2½-pound (2-inch thick) tri-tip
- 1 teaspoon liquid smoke
- 1 tablespoon extra-virgin olive oil

Directions:

1.   Attach the sous vide immersion circulator to a Cambro container or pot with water using an adjustable clamp and preheat water to 135°F.

2.   In a bowl, combine garlic salt and black pepper. Sprinkle tri-tip with garlic salt mixture generously.

3.   Place tri-tip, liquid smoke, and oil in a cooking pouch. Seal pouch tightly after removing the excess air. Place pouch in sous vide bath and set the cooking time for 2 hours.

4.   Preheat grill to high heat.

5.   Remove pouch from the sous vide bath and open carefully. Remove tri-tip from pouch and pat dry with paper towels.

6.   Grill tri-tip for 1 minute on each side.

7.   Remove from grill and cut into desired slices. Serve immediately.

Pork Chops With Mushroom Sauce

Servings: 3

Cooking Time: 1 Hour 10 Minutes

Ingredients:

- 3 (8 oz) pork chops
- Salt and black pepper to taste
- 3 tbsp butter, unsalted
- 6 oz mushrooms
- ½ cup beef stock
- 2 tbsp Worcestershire sauce
- 3 tbsp garlic chives, chopped for garnishing

Directions:

1.   Make a water bath, place Sous Vide in it, and set to 140 F. Rub pork chops with salt and pepper and place in a vacuum-sealable bag. Release air by the

water displacement method, seal and submerge the bag in the water bath. Set the timer for 55 minutes.

2. Once the timer has stopped, remove and unseal the bag. Remove the pork and pat dry using a paper towel. Discard the juices. Place a skillet over medium heat and add 1 tablespoon butter. Sear pork for 2 minutes on both sides. Set aside. With the skillet still over the heat, add the mushrooms and cook for 5 minutes. Turn heat off, add in the remaining butter and swirl until butter melts. Season with pepper and salt. Serve pork chops with mushroom sauce over it.

Sweet Mustard Pork With Crispy Onions

Servings: 6
Cooking Time: 48 Hours 40 Minutes
Ingredients:
- 1 tbsp ketchup
- 4 tbsp honey mustard
- 2 tbsp soy sauce
- 2¼ pounds pork shoulder
- 1 large sweet onion, cut into thin rings
- 2 cups milk
- 1½ cups all-purpose flour
- 2 tsp granulated onion powder
- 1 tsp paprika
- Salt and black pepper to taste
- 4 cups vegetable oil, for frying

Directions:
1. Prepare a water bath and place the Sous Vide in it. Set to 159 F.
2. Combine well the mustard, soy sauce and ketchup to make a paste. Brush the pork with the sauce and place in a vacuum-sealable bag. Release air by the water displacement method, seal and submerge the bag in the water bath. Cook for 48 hours.
3. To make the onions: separate the onion rings in a bowl. Pour the milk over them and allow to chill for 1 hour. Combine the flour, onion powder paprika, and a pinch of salt and pepper.
4. Heat the oil in a skillet to 375 F. Drain the onions and deepen in the flour mix. Shake well and transfer into the skillet. Fry them for 2 minutes or until gets crispy. Transfer to a baking sheet and pat dry with

kitchen towel. Repeat the process with the remaining onions.

5. Once the timer has stopped, remove the pork and transfer to a cutting board and pull the pork until it is shredded. Reserve cooking juices and transfer into a saucepan hot over medium heat and cook for 5 minutes until reduced. Top the pork with the sauce and garnish with the crispy onions to serve.

Beef Wellington

Servings: 6
Cooking Time: 1hr. 15min
Ingredients:
- ½ beef tenderloin, unsliced, silver skin removed
- 1 teaspoon salt
- 1 teaspoon pepper
- ¼ pound prosciutto, sliced thin
- ½ cup mushrooms, minced
- 1 shallot, minced
- ½ tablespoon tomato paste
- 2 tablespoons butter, softened
- 1 sheet refrigerated puff pastry
- 1 egg, beaten

Directions:
1. Preheat the sous vide bath to 140 degrees F. Season the beef to taste then add to a vacuum seal bag. Seal, and cook in bath for about an hour. Set in the refrigerator. Sauté shallots in butter until translucent, then add mushrooms and sauté until cooked. Pour into a bowl and stir in tomato paste.
2. When the beef has cooled completely, preheat oven to 400 degrees F. Lay puff pastry on a cutting board and spread a layer of prosciutto on top. Place the chilled beef on top of the puff pastry and spread the duxelles on all sides of the beef. Wrap the prosciutto-lined pastry around the beef and seal with egg. Brush remaining egg over pastry to glaze.
3. Bake beef Wellington 15 minutes or until puff pastry is golden-brown and fully cooked. Slice across the grain to serve.
Nutrition Info: Calories: 649 Protein: 448gCarbs: 49gFat: 101g

Sirloin Steak With Smashed Yukon Potatoes

Servings: 4
Cooking Time: 60 Minutes
Ingredients:

- 4 sirloin steaks
- 2 lbs. baby Yukon potatoes, cubed
- ¼ cup steak seasoning
- Salt and pepper as needed
- 4 tablespoon butter
- Canola oil for searing

Directions:

1. Prepare the Sous Vide water bath using your immersion circulator and raise the temperature to 129-degrees Fahrenheit
2. Season the steaks. Seal the steaks in a zip bag using the immersion method and cook for 1 hour
3. Take the potatoes and cook them in boiling water for 15 minutes
4. Strain the potatoes into a large mixing bowl and add the butter. Mash using the back of your spoon until mixed well
5. Season with salt and pepper
6. Once cooked, take the steak out from the bag and pat it dry using a kitchen towel
7. Heat a heavy bottomed pan over medium-heat and add the oil. Sear the steak for 1 minute
8. Serve with the smashed potatoes

Nutrition Info: Per serving:Calories: 473 ;Carbohydrate: 32g ;Protein: 30g ;Fat: 27g ;Sugar: 5g ;Sodium: 546mg

Asian-style Pork With Rice & Ginger

Servings: 4
Cooking Time: 2 Hours 10 Minutes
Ingredients:

- 1 cup brown rice
- 8 cups chicken stock
- 1 pound ground pork
- 1 tbsp minced fresh ginger
- 1 tsp minced fresh garlic
- 1 tbsp coconut oil
- 1 cup basil chiffonade
- Salt and black pepper to taste

Directions:

1. Prepare a water bath and place the Sous Vide in it. Set to 192 F. Place the rice in a vacuum-sealable bag. Release air by the water displacement method, seal and submerge the bag in the water bath. Cook for 1 hour and 30 minutes.
2. Once the timer has stopped, remove the rice and season with salt and pepper. Heat a skillet over medium heat and cook the pork, garlic and ginger. Remove from the heat and put basil. Season with salt and pepper. Serve the rice in bowls with the ginger pork mix.

Drunken Beef Steak

Servings: 4
Cooking Time: 2 Hours 15 Minutes
Ingredients:

- 1 pound beef steak
- 1 cup red wine
- 2 tsp butter
- 1 tsp sugar
- Salt and black pepper to taste

Directions:

1. Prepare a water bath and place the Sous Vide in it. Set to 131 F. Combine red wine with the spices and pour into a vacuum-sealable bag. Place the meat inside.Release air by the water displacement method, seal and submerge the bag in water bath. Set the timer for 2 hours. Once the timer has stopped, remove the bag. Melt butter in a pan and sear the meat on all sides for a few minutes.

Jerk Pork Ribs

Servings: 6
Cooking Time: 20 Hours 10 Minutes
Ingredients:

- 5 lb (2) baby back pork ribs, full racks
- ½ cup jerk seasoning mix

Directions:

1. Make a water bath, place Sous Vide in it, and set to 145 F. Cut the racks into halves and season them with half of jerk seasoning. Place the racks in separate vacuum-sealable racks. Release air by the water displacement method, seal and submerge the bags in the water bath. Set the timer to 20 hours.

2. Cover the water bath with a bag to reduce evaporation and add water every 3 hours to avoid the water drying out. Once the timer has stopped, remove and unseal the bag. Transfer the ribs to a foiled baking sheet and preheat a broiler to high. Rub the ribs with the remaining jerk seasoning and place them in the broiler. Broil for 5 minutes. Slice into single ribs.

Beef & Veggie Stew

Servings: 12
Cooking Time: 4 Hours 25 Minutes
Ingredients:
- 16 ounces beef fillet, cubed
- 4 potatoes, chopped
- 3 carrots, sliced
- 5 ounces shallot, sliced
- 1 onion, chopped
- 2 garlic cloves, minced
- ¼ cup red wine
- ¼ cup heavy cream
- 2 tbsp butter
- 1 tsp paprika
- ½ cup chicken stock
- ½ tsp turmeric
- Salt and black pepper to taste
- 1 tsp lemon juice

Directions:
1. Prepare a water bath and place the Sous Vide in it. Set to 155 F. Place the beef along with salt, pepper, turmeric, paprika, and red wine in a vacuum-sealable bag. Massage to coat well. Release air by the water displacement method, seal and submerge the bag in water bath. Set the timer for 4 hours.
2. Meanwhile, combine the remaining ingredients in another vacuum-sealable bag. Seal and immerse it in the same bath 3 hours before the end of the cooking time of the meat. Once done, remove everything and place in a pot over medium heat and cook for 15 minutes.

Osso Buco

Cooking Time: 72 Hours 15 Mins Cooking
Temperature: 143°f

Ingredients:
- 2 veal shanks
- salt and freshly ground black pepper, to taste
- flour, as required
- extra-virgin olive oil, as required
- butter, as required
- 1 onion, chopped
- 2 ounces pancetta, chopped
- 1 glass dry white wine
- ½ cup concentrated veal broth
- 2 teaspoons tomato paste
- For Gremolata:
- fresh flat leaf parsley, as required
- 1 fresh sprig rosemary
- 2 fresh sage leaves
- fresh lemon zest, as required
- 1 garlic clove

Directions:
1. Attach the sous vide immersion circulator using an adjustable clamp to a Cambro container or pot filled with water and preheat to 143°F.
2. With a sharp knife, make 1-inch cuts in the around the shanks.
3. With paper towels, pat shanks and season with salt and black pepper.
4. Dust each shank with flour evenly.
5. In a frying pan, heat olive oil and sear shanks until browned from both sides.
6. Transfer shanks onto a plate. Discard most of the oil from the pan.
7. In the same pan, melt butter and sauté onion until translucent.
8. Add pancetta and sauté until slightly golden.
9. Stir in wine and cook until half the wine is absorbed.
10. Stir in veal broth and tomato paste, then remove from heat.
11. Into a large cooking ouch, place shanks and wine mixture. Seal pouch tightly after squeezing out the excess air. Place pouch in sous vide bath and set the cooking time for 72 hours.
12. Meanwhile for gremolata:
13. in a food processor, add all ingredients listed under gremolata section above, and pulse until minced finely.

14. Remove pouch from sous vide bath and carefully open it. Remove shanks from pouch.

15. Transfer shanks with mixture onto serving platter. Top with gremolata and serve.

Lemony & Peppery Flank Steak

Servings: 4
Cooking Time: 2 Hours 15 Minutes
Ingredients:
- 2 pounds flank steak
- 1 tbsp lime zest
- 1 lemon, sliced
- ½ tsp cayenne pepper
- 1 tsp garlic powder
- Salt and black pepper to taste
- ¼ cup maple syrup
- ½ cup chicken stock

Directions:
1. Prepare a water bath and place the Sous Vide in it. Set to 148 F. Combine the spices and zest and rub over the steak. Let sit for about 5 minutes.
2. Whisk the stock and maple syrup. Place the steak in a vacuum-sealable bag and add the lemon slices. Release air by the water displacement method, seal and submerge the bag in water bath. Set timer for 2 hours. Once done, remove and transfer to a grill and cook for 30 seconds each side. Serve immediately.

Minted Lamb Chops With Nuts

Servings: 4
Cooking Time: 2 Hours 35 Minutes
Ingredients:
- 1 pound lamb chops
- Salt and black pepper to taste
- 1 cup fresh mint leaves
- ½ cup cashew nuts
- ½ cup packed fresh parsley
- ½ cup scallion, sliced
- 3 tbsp lemon juice
- 2 cloves garlic, minced
- 6 tbsp olive oil

Directions:

1. Prepare a water bath and place the Sous Vide in it. Set to 125 F. Season the lamb with salt and pepper and place in a vacuum-sealable bag. Release air by the water displacement method, seal and submerge the bag in water bath. Cook for 2 hours.
2. In a food processor blend the mint, parsley, cashews, scallions, garlic, and lemon juice. Pour 4 tbsp of olive oil. Season with salt and pepper. Once the timer has stopped, remove the lamb, brush with 2 tbsp of olive oil and transfer to a hot grill. Cook for 1 minute per side. Serve with nuts.

Spicy Tenderloin

Servings: 4
Cooking Time: 3 Hours 15 Minutes
Ingredients:
- 1 pound pork tenderloin, trimmed
- Salt to taste
- ½ tsp black pepper
- 3 tbsp chili paste

Directions:
1. Prepare a water bath and place the Sous Vide in it. Set to 146 F.
2. Combine the tenderloin with salt and pepper and place in a vacuum-sealable bag. Release air by the water displacement method, seal and submerge the bag in the water bath. Cook for 3 hours.
3. Once the timer has stopped, remove the pork and brush with chili paste. Heat a grill over high heat and sear the tenderloin for 5 minutes until browned. Allow resting. Cut the tenderloin into slices and serve.

Venison Steaks

Cooking Time: 36 Hours Cooking Temperature: 137°f
Ingredients:
- For Steaks:
- 1 x 1-pound venison blade steak
- 2 shallots, roughly chopped
- 6 cloves garlic, roughly chopped
- 3 chili peppers, seeded and roughly chopped
- salt and freshly ground black pepper, to taste
- 1 tablespoon avocado oil
- For Gravy:
- reserved cooking liquid mixture

- 2 tablespoons butter
- 1 teaspoon all-purpose flour
- 1 cup beef broth
- For Garnish:
- black mustard blossoms
- micro green herbs
- red amaranth

Directions:
1. For the steak:
2. to a large bowl, add the steak, shallots, garlic, chili peppers, salt, and pepper, and and toss to coat well.
3. Refrigerate for at least 30 minutes.
4. Attach the sous vide immersion circulator using an adjustable clamp to a Cambro container.or pot filled with water and preheat to 137°F.
5. Into a cooking pouch, add steak mixture. Seal pouch tightly after squeezing out the excess air. Place pouch in sous vide bath and place a weight over pouch. Set the cooking time for 36 hours.
6. Remove pouch from sous vide bath and carefully open it. Remove steak from pouch, reserving cooking liquid mixture. With paper towels, pat steak completely dry and set aside to rest briefly.
7. In a skillet, heat 1 tablespoon of avocado oil and sear steak for 1 minute per side.
8. Transfer steak onto a plate and keep aside.
9. For the gravy:
10. in in a food processor, add the reserved cooking liquid mixture and pulse until a smooth paste is formed.
11. In a heavy-bottomed pan, melt butter. Stir in flour and paste cook until browned slightly, stirring continuously.
12. Reduce heat and stir in paste and broth. Bring to a boil and remove from heat.
13. Cut steak into desired slices and decorate with favorite garnish.
14. Serve with gravy.

Prime Rib

Servings: 12
Cooking Time: 6 Hours
Ingredients:
- 3 lbs. bone-in beef ribeye roast

- Kosher salt as needed
- 1 tablespoon black peppercorn, coarsely ground
- 1 tablespoon green peppercorn, coarsely ground
- 1 tablespoon pink peppercorn, coarsely ground
- 1 tablespoon dried celery seeds
- 2 tablespoons dried garlic powder
- 4 sprigs rosemary
- 1-quart beef stock
- 2 egg whites

Directions:
1. Season the beef with kosher salt and chill for 12 hours
2. Prepare the Sous Vide water bath using your immersion circulator and raise the temperature to 132-degrees Fahrenheit
3. Add the beef in a zip bag and seal using the immersion method. Cook for 6 hours
4. Pre-heat the oven to 425-degrees Fahrenheit and remove the beef. Pat it dry
5. Mix the peppercorns, celery seeds, garlic powder and rosemary together in a bowl
6. Brush the top of your cooked roast with egg white and season with the mixture and salt
7. Put the roast on a baking rack and roast for 10-15 minutes. Allow it to rest for 10-15 minutes and carve
8. Pour the cooking liquid from the bag in a large saucepan, bring to a boil and simmer until the amount has halved.
9. Carve the roast and serve with the stock.

Nutrition Info: Per serving:Calories: 504 ;Carbohydrate: 4g ;Protein: 33g ;Fat: 40g ;Sugar: 0g ;Sodium: 1025mg

Kimchi Rib Eye Tacos With Avocado

Servings: 4
Cooking Time: 2 Hours 25 Minutes
Ingredients:
- 2 pounds short rib, thinly sliced
- ½ cup soy sauce
- 3 green onion stalks, sliced
- 1 tbsp Tabasco sauce
- 6 cloves garlic, chopped
- 2 tbsp brown sugar
- 1-inch turmeric, grated

- 1 tbsp sesame oil
- ½ a tsp red pepper powder
- 8 corn tortillas
- Kimchi for topping
- 1 Sliced avocado

Directions:

1. Prepare a water bath and place the Sous Vide in it. Set to 138 F.

2. Heat a saucepan over medium heat and combine soy sauce, green onion, garlic, tabasco sauce, brown sugar, turmeric, red pepper powder, and sesame oil. Cook until the sugar dissolved. Allow chilling.

3. Place the sauce mixture in a vacuum-sealable bag. Release air by the water displacement method, seal and submerge the bag in the water bath. Cook for 2 hours. Once the timer has stopped, remove the sauce and transfer to a saucepan for reduced. In a grill, put the short ribs and cook until crispy. Chop the ribs in cubes. Create a taco with the tortilla, beef and avocado. Garnish with Kimchi and hot sauce.

Fire-roasted Tomato Tenderloin

Servings: 4

Cooking Time: 2 Hours 8 Minutes

Ingredients:

- 2 pounds center-cut beef tenderloin, 1-inch thick
- 1 cup fire-roasted tomatoes, chopped
- Salt and black pepper to taste
- 3 tbsp of extra virgin olive oil
- 2 bay leaves, whole
- 3 tbsp of butter, unsalted

Directions:

1. Prepare a water bath, place Sous Vide in it, and set to 136 F. Thoroughly rinse the meat under the running water and pat dry with paper towels. Rub well with the olive oil and generously season with salt and pepper. Place in a large vacuum-sealable bag along with fire-roasted tomatoes and two bay leaves. Seal the bag, submerge in the water bath and cook for 2 hours.

2. Once done, remove the bags, place the meat on a baking sheet. Discard the cooking liquid. In a large skillet, melt the butter over medium heat. Add the tenderloin and sear for 2 minutes on each side. Serve with your favorite sauce and vegetables.

Easy-to-make Tenderloin With Cayenne Sauce

Servings: 2

Cooking Time: 55 Minutes

Ingredients:

- 16 beef tenderloin steaks
- ¼ tsp cayenne powder
- Salt and black pepper to taste
- ½ tbsp butter
- ½ tbsp olive oil
- 2 tbsp onion, finely chopped
- 1 clove garlic, minced
- ¼ cup sherry
- 2 tbsp balsamic vinegar
- 1 chipotle pepper
- ¼ cup water
- 1 tbsp tomato paste
- 1 tsp soy sauce
- 1 tbsp molasses
- 1 tbsp vegetable oil
- Cilantro, chopped, for garnish

Directions:

1. Prepare a water bath and place the Sous Vide in it. Set to 125 F.

2. Combine the steak with chipotle pepper, salt and pepper, and place in a vacuum-sealable bag. Release air by the water displacement method, seal and submerge the bag in water bath. Cook for 40 minutes.

3. Meanwhile, prepare the sauce by heating a skillet over medium heat. Add in butter and onion, and cook until softened. Stir in garlic and cook for 1 more minute. Pour in sherry and cook until reduced. Pour in balsamic vinegar, cayenne, water, tomato paste, soy sauce, and molasses. Stir. Broil until thick.

4. Once the timer has stopped, remove the steak and transfer to a heated skillet with butter over high heat and sear for 1 minute. Top with the sauce and garnish with cilantro to serve.

Dijon & Curry Ketchup Beef Sausages

Servings: 4

Cooking Time: 1 Hour 45 Minutes

Ingredients:

- ½ cup Dijon mustard
- 4 beef sausages
- ½ cup curry ketchup

Directions:

1. Prepare a water bath and place the Sous Vide in it. Set to 134 F.
2. Place the sausages in a vacuum-sealable bag. Release air by the water displacement method, seal and submerge the bag in the water bath. Cook for 90 minutes. Once the timer has stopped, remove the sausages and transfer to a high heat grill. Cook for 1-3 minutes until the grill marks appear. Serve with the mustard and curry ketchup.

Lamb Shank With Veggies & Sweet Sauce

Servings: 4
Cooking Time: 48 Hours 45 Minutes
Ingredients:

- 4 lamb shanks
- 2 tbsp oil
- 2 cups all-purpose flour
- 1 red onion, sliced
- 4 garlic cloves, smashed and peeled
- 4 carrots, medium diced
- 4 stalks celery, medium diced
- 3 tbsp tomato paste
- ½ cup sherry wine vinegar
- 1 cup red wine
- ¾ cup honey
- 1 cup beef stock
- 4 sprigs fresh rosemary
- 2 bay leaves
- Salt and black pepper to taste

Directions:

1. Prepare a water bath and place the Sous Vide in it. Set to 155 F.
2. Heat oil in a skillet over high heat. Season the shanks with salt, pepper and flour. Sear until golden brown. Set aside. Reduce the heat and cook the onion, carrots, garlic, and celery for 10 minutes. Season with salt and pepper. Stir in tomato paste and cook for 1 more minute. Add in vinegar, stock, wine, honey, bay leaves. Cook for 2 minutes.

3. Place the veggies, sauce and lambs in a vacuum-sealable bag. Release air by the water displacement method, seal and submerge the bag in the water bath. Cook for 48 hours.
4. Once the timer has stopped, remove the shanks and dry it. Reserve the cooking juices. Sear the shanks for 5 minutes until golden. Heat a saucepan over high and pour in cooking juices. Cook until reduced, for 10 minutes. Transfer the shanks to a plate and drizzle with the sauce to serve.

Standing Rib Roast

Cooking Time: 24-36 Hours Cooking Temperature: 130°f
Ingredients:

- 1 x 3-rib standing rib roast (6-8 pounds) (a.k.a. prime rib roast)
- 1-2 ounces dried morel mushrooms
- kosher salt and freshly cracked black pepper, to taste
- 3 ounces garlic-infused olive oil

Directions:

1. Attach the sous vide immersion circulator using an adjustable clamp to a Cambro container or pot filled with water and preheat to 130°F.
2. Into a cooking pouch, add rib roast and mushrooms. Seal pouch tightly after squeezing out the excess air. Place pouch in sous vide bath and set the cooking time for at least 24 and up to 36 hours.
3. Remove pouch from sous vide bath and carefully open it. Transfer rib roast onto a cutting board, reserving mushroom and cooking liquid into a bowl. With paper towels, pat rib roast completely dry.
4. Rub rib roast with salt and black pepper evenly.
5. Heat cast iron pan to medium high heat and place the rib roast in, fat cap down. Sear for 1-2 minutes per side (or until browned on all sides).
6. Meanwhile, season reserved mushroom mixture with garlic oil, a little salt, and black pepper.
7. Transfer rib roast onto a cutting board, bone side down.
8. Carefully, remove rib bones and cut rib roast into ½-inch-thick slices across the grain.
9. Serve immediately with mushroom mixture.

Greek Meatballs With Yogurt Sauce

Servings: 4
Cooking Time: 1 Hour 10 Minutes
Ingredients:

- 1 pound lean ground beef
- ¼ cup bread crumbs
- 1 large egg, beaten
- 2 teaspons fresh parsley
- Sea salt and black pepper to taste
- 3 tbsp extra-virgin olive oil
- Yogurt Sauce:
- 6 ounces Greek yogurt
- 1 tbsp extra-virgin olive oil
- Fresh dill
- Lemon juice from 1 lemon
- 1 garlic clove, minced
- Salt to taste

Directions:

1. Start with the preparation of yougurt sauce. Whisk together all sauce ingredients in a medium bowl, cover and refrigerate for a 1 hour.
2. Now, prepare a water bath, place Sous Vide in it, and set to 141 F. Place the meat in a large bowl. Add the beaten egg, bread crumbs, fresh parsley, salt, and pepper. Thoroughly combine the ingredients together. Shape bite-sized balls and place in a large vacuum-sealable bag in a single layer. Seal the bag and cook in a water bath for 1 hour. With a slotted spoon carefully remove from the bag and discard the cooking liquid.
3. Sear the meatballs in a medium-hot skillet with olive oil until they are browned, 2-3 minutes per side. Top with yogurt sauce and serve.

Mango Salsa & Pork

Servings: 4
Cooking Time: 2 Hours
Ingredients:

- ¼ cup light broth sugar
- 1 tablespoon ground allspice
- ½ teaspoon cayenne pepper
- ¼ teaspoon ground cinnamon
- ¼ teaspoon ground cloves
- Kosher salt and black pepper, as needed

- 2 lbs. pork tenderloin
- 2 tablespoons canola oil
- 2 pitted and peeled mangoes, finely diced
- ¼ cup fresh cilantro, chopped
- 1 red bell pepper, stemmed, seeded, and finely diced
- 3 tablespoons red onion, finely diced
- 2 tablespoons freshly squeezed lime juice
- 1 small jalapeno seeded and finely diced

Directions:

1. Prepare the Sous Vide water bath using your immersion circulator and raise the temperature to 135-degrees Fahrenheit.
2. Take a medium bowl and mix the sugar, allspice, cinnamon, cayenne, cloves, 2 teaspoons of salt, and 1 teaspoon of pepper.
3. Rub the mixture over the tenderloins.
4. Take a large-sized skillet and put it over medium heat, add the oil and once the oil simmers, transfer the pork and sear for 5 minutes, browning all sides.
5. Transfer to a plate and rest for 10 minutes.
6. Transfer the pork chop to a resealable zipper bag and seal using the immersion method. Cook for 2 hours.
7. Once cooked, take the bag out and allow it to rest for a while, take the chop out and slice it.
8. Prepare the salsa by mixing the mango, cilantro, bell pepper, onion, lime juice, and jalapeno in a mixing bowl.
9. Serve the sliced pork with salsa with a seasoning salt and pepper.

Nutrition Info: Per serving:Calories: 217 ;Carbohydrate: 11g ;Protein: 25g ;Fat: 8g ;Sugar: 8g ;Sodium: 112mg

Herb Crusted Lamb Rack

Servings: 6
Cooking Time: 3 Hours 30 Minutes
Ingredients:

- Lamb Rack:
- 3 large racks of lamb
- Salt and black pepper to taste
- 1 sprig rosemary
- 2 tbsp olive oil
- Herb Crust:

- 2 tbsp fresh rosemary leaves
- ½ cup macadamia nuts
- 2 tbsp Dijon mustard
- ½ cup fresh parsley
- 2 tbsp fresh thyme leaves
- 2 tbsp lemon zest
- 2 cloves garlic
- 2 Egg whites

Directions:

1. Make a water bath, place the Sous Vide in it, and set to 140 F.
2. Pat dry the lamb using a paper towel and rub the meat with salt and black pepper. Place a pan over medium heat and add in olive oil. Once heated, sear the lamb on both sides for 2 minutes; set aside.
3. Place in garlic and rosemary, toast for 2 minutes and place the lamb over. Let lamb absorb the flavors for 5 minutes.
4. Place lamb, garlic, and rosemary in a vacuum-sealable bag, release air by the water displacement method and seal the bag. Submerge the bag in the water bath.
5. Set the timer to cook for 3 hours. Once the timer has stopped, remove the bag, unseal it and take out the lamb. Whisk the egg whites and set aside.
6. Blend the remaining listed herb crust ingredients using a blender and set aside. Pat dry the lamb using a paper towel and brush with the egg whites. Dip into the herb mixture and coat graciously.
7. Place the lamb racks with crust side up on a baking sheet. Bake in an oven for 15 minutes. Gently slice each cutlet using a sharp knife. Serve with a side of pureed vegetables.

Sweet Orange Pork Tacos

Servings: 8
Cooking Time: 7 Hours 10 Minutes
Ingredients:

- ½ cup orange juice
- 4 tbsp honey
- 2 tbsp fresh garlic, minced
- 2 tbsp fresh ginger, minced
- 2 tbsp Worcestershire sauce
- 2 tsp hoisin sauce
- 2 tsp sriracha sauce
- Zest of ½ orange
- 1 pound pork shoulder
- 8 flour tortillas, warmed
- ½ cup chopped fresh cilantro
- 1 lime, cut into wedges

Directions:

1. Prepare a water bath and place the Sous Vide in it. Set to 175 F.
2. Combine well the orange juice, 3 tbsp of honey, garlic, ginger, Worcestershire sauce, hoisin sauce, sriracha, and orange zest.
3. Place the pork in a vacuum-sealable bag, and add in orange sauce. Release air by the water displacement method, seal and submerge the bag in the water bath. Cook for 7 hours.
4. Once the timer has stopped, remove the pork and transfer to a baking sheet. Reserve cooking juices.
5. Heat a saucepan over medium heat and pour in juices with the remaining honey. Cook for 5 minutes until bubbling and reduced by half. Brush the pork with the sauce. Fill the tortillas with the pork. Garnish with cilantro and top with the remaining sauce to serve.

Sherry Braised Pork Ribs

Servings: 4
Cooking Time: 18 Hours 10 Minutes
Ingredients:

- 2 pounds pork ribs, chopped into bone sections
- 1 tbsp ginger root, sliced
- ½ tsp ground nutmeg
- 2 tbsp soy sauce
- 1 tsp salt
- 1 tsp white sugar
- 1 anise star pod
- ¼ cup dry sherry
- 1 tbsp butter

Directions:

1. In a small bowl, combine salt, sugar and ground nutmeg, and rub the pork ribs with this mixture.
2. Put the ribs into the vacuum bag, add sliced ginger root, soy sauce, anise star and sherry wine.
3. Preheat your sous vide machine to 176ºF.
4. Set the cooking time for 18 hours.

5. When the time is up, carefully dry the ribs with the paper towels.

6. Sear the ribs in 1 tbsp butter on both sides for about 40 seconds until crusty.

Nutrition Info: Per serving:Calories 284, Carbohydrates 32 g, Fats 12 g, Protein 12 g

Pork & Bean Stew

Servings: 8

Cooking Time: 7 Hours 20 Minutes

Ingredients:
- 2 tbsp vegetable oil
- 1 tbsp butter
- 1 trimmed pork loin, cubed
- Salt and black pepper to taste
- 2 cups frozen pearl onions
- 2 large parsnips, chopped
- 2 minced cloves garlic
- 2 tbsp all-purpose flour
- 1 cup dry white wine
- 2 cups chicken stock
- 1 can white beans, drained and rinsed
- 4 fresh rosemary sprigs
- 2 bay leaves

Directions:

1. Prepare a water bath and place the Sous Vide in it. Set to 138 F.

2. Heat a non-stick pan over high heat with butter and oil. Add the pork. Season with pepper and salt. Cook for 7 minutes. Put in onions and cook for 5 minutes. Mix the garlic and wine until bubble. Stir in beans, rosemary, stock, and bay leaves. Remove from the heat.

3. Place the pork in a vacuum-sealable bag. Release air by the water displacement method, seal and submerge the bag in the water bath. Cook for 7 hours. Once the timer has stopped, remove the bag and transfer into a bowl. Garnish with rosemary.

Venison Shoulder

Cooking Time: 8 Hours 15 Mins Cooking

Temperature: 130°f

Ingredients:
- farmed venison bolar roast *

- salt and freshly ground black pepper, to taste
- clarified butter *
- red wine *
- cold butter, cut into small pieces *

Directions:

1. Attach the sous vide immersion circulator using an adjustable clamp to a Cambro container or pot filled with water and preheat to 130°F.

2. Season roast evenly with salt and black pepper.

3. Into a cooking pouch, add roast. Seal pouch tightly after squeezing out the excess air. Place pouch in sous vide bath and set the cooking time for 8 hours.

4. Remove pouch from sous vide bath and carefully open it. Remove venison loin from pouch, reserving pouch juices. With paper towels, pat roast completely dry.

5. In a skillet, melt clarified butter over a very high heat, and sear roast for 1 minute per side.

6. Remove from skillet and transfer onto a cutting board to rest. Cover roast with a piece of foil to keep warm.

7. Add reserved juices into a small pan and bring to a boil.

8. To the skillet used for the roast, add red wine and, using a wooden spatula, scrape the browned pieces from bottom and sides.

9. Strain reserved juices from the sous vide pouch into pan and bring to a boil. Cook until sauce is cooked to taste.

10. Reduce heat to very low. Add cold butter and cook until mixture becomes slightly thick, beating continuously.

11. Cut roast into slices across the grain. Serve roast slices with butter sauce.

Red Wine Beef Ribs

Servings: 3

Cooking Time: 6 Hours 15 Minutes

Ingredients:
- 1 pound beef short ribs
- ¼ cup red wine
- 1 tsp honey
- ½ cup tomato paste
- 2 tbsp olive oil
- ½ cup beef stock

- ¼ cup apple cider vinegar
- 1 garlic clove, minced
- 1 tsp Paprika
- Salt and black pepper to taste

Directions:

1. Prepare a water bath and place the Sous Vide in it. Set to 140 F. Rinse and drain the ribs. Season with salt, pepper, and paprika. Place in a vacuum-sealable bag in a single layer along with wine, tomato paste, beef broth, honey, and apple cider. Release air by the water displacement method, seal and submerge the bag in the water bath. Set the timer for 6 hours. Pat the ribs dry. Discard cooking liquids.

2. In a large skillet, heat up the olive oil over medium heat. Add garlic and stir-fry until translucent. Put in ribs and brown for 5 minutes per side.

Classic Cheese Burgers

Servings: 4
Cooking Time: 1 Hour 15 Minutes
Ingredients:

- 1 pound ground beef
- 2 hamburger buns
- 2 slices cheddar cheese
- Salt and black pepper to taste
- Butter for toasting

Directions:

1. Prepare a water bath and place the Sous Vide in it. Set to 137 F. Season beef with salt and pepper and shape into patties. Place in a vacuum-sealable bag. Release air by the water displacement method, seal and submerge the bag in the water bath. Cook for 1 hour.

2. Meanwhile, heat a skillet and toast the buns with butter. Once the timer has stopped, remove the burgers and transfer to a skillet. Sear for 30 seconds per side. Top the burger with cheese and cook until melted. Put the burger between the buns and serve.

Sweet Spare Ribs With Mango Soy Sauce

Servings: 4
Cooking Time: 36 Hours 25 Minutes
Ingredients:

- 4 pounds pork spare ribs

- Salt and black pepper to taste
- 1 cup mango juice
- ¼ cup soy sauce
- 3 tbsp honey
- 1 tbsp chili garlic paste
- 1 tbsp ground ginger
- 2 tbsp coconut oil
- 1 tsp Chinese five-spice powder
- 1 tsp ground coriander

Directions:

1. Prepare a water bath and place the Sous Vide in it. Set to 146 F.

2. Season the ribs with salt and pepper and place in a vacuum-sealable bag. Release air by the water displacement method, seal and submerge the bag in the water bath. Cook for 36 hours. Once the timer has stopped, remove the ribs and pat dry. Discard cooking juices.

3. Heat a saucepan over medium heat and boil mango juice, soy sauce, chili, garlic paste, honey, ginger, coconut oil, five-spices, and coriander for 10 minutes until reduced. Drizzle the ribs with the sauce. Transfer to a baking tray and cook for 5 minutes in the oven at 390 F.

Cream-poached Pork Loin

Servings: 4
Cooking Time: 4 Hours
Ingredients:

- 1 – 3 lbs. boneless pork loin roast
- Kosher salt and pepper as needed
- 2 thinly sliced onion
- ¼ cup cognac
- 1 cup whole milk
- 1 cup heavy cream

Directions:

1. Prepare the Sous Vide water bath using your immersion circulator and raise the temperature to 145-degrees Fahrenheit.

2. Season the pork with pepper and salt, take a large iron skillet and place it over medium-heat for 5 minutes.

3. Add the pork and sear for 15 minutes until all sides are browned.

4. Transfer to a platter, add the onion to the rendered fat (in the skillet) and cook for 5 minutes.
5. Add the cognac and bring to a simmer. Allow it to cool for 10 minutes.
6. Add the pork, onion, milk, and cream to a resealable zipper bag and seal using the immersion method. Submerge underwater and cook for 4 hours.
7. Once cooked, remove the bag from the water and take the pork out, transfer the pork to cutting board and cover it to keep it warm.
8. Pour the bag contents to a skillet and bring the mixture to a simmer over medium heat, keep cooking for 10 minutes and season with salt and pepper.
9. Slice the pork and serve with the cream sauce.

Nutrition Info: Per serving:Calories: 1809 ;Carbohydrate: 23g ;Protein: 109g ;Fat: 140g ;Sugar: 19g ;Sodium: 621mg

Beef Tenderloin With Lemon Parsley Butter

Cooking Time: 1-4 Hours Cooking Temperature: 140°f

Ingredients:
- 1½-pound center cut beef tenderloin, trimmed
- Kosher salt and freshly cracked black pepper, to taste
- 4 thyme sprigs
- 7 tablespoons unsalted butter, softened and divided
- 1 garlic clove, minced
- 2 tablespoons fresh parsley leaves, chopped
- 1 teaspoon fresh lemon zest
- 1 teaspoon fresh lemon juice
- 1 tablespoon vegetable oil

Directions:
1. Attach the sous vide immersion circulator to a Cambro container or pot with water using an adjustable clamp and preheat water to 140°F.
2. With a sharp knife, cut tenderloin into 4 6-ounce portions. Place each portion onto a cutting board, cut-side down and flatten gently with your hand until the portion reaches 2-inch thickness. Season tenderloin generously with salt and black pepper.
3. Place beef tenderloin and thyme sprigs in a cooking pouch. Seal pouch tightly after removing the excess air. Place pouch in sous vide bath and set the cooking time for a minimum of 1 hour and a maximum time of 4 hours.
4. While tenderloin cooks, combine 6 tablespoons of butter, garlic, parsley, lemon zest, lemon juice, salt, and black pepper in a bowl. Set aside.
5. Remove pouch from the sous vide bath and open carefully. Remove tenderloin pieces from pouch and pat dry with paper towels.
6. In a heavy-bottomed 12-inch skillet, heat oil and remaining butter over high heat and sear tenderloin pieces for 1 minute on each side.
7. Divide tenderloin pieces onto serving plates. Top with parsley butter and serve immediately.

Beef Sirloin In Tomato Sauce

Servings: 3
Cooking Time: 2 Hours 5 Minutes
Ingredients:
- 1 pound beef sirloin medallions
- 1 cup fire-roasted tomatoes
- 1 tsp hot pepper sauce
- 3 garlic cloves, crushed
- 2 tsp chili pepper
- 2 tsp garlic powder
- 2 tsp fresh lime juice
- 1 bay leaf
- 2 tsp vegetable oil
- Salt and black pepper to taste

Directions:
1. Prepare a water bath, place Sous Vide in it, and set to 129 F. Season beef with salt and black pepper.
2. In a bowl, combine the fire roasted tomatoes with hot pepper sauce, crushed garlic, chili pepper, garlic powder, and lime juice. Add the sirloin to the mixture and toss to coat. Place in the vacuum-sealable bag in a single layer and seal it. Submerge in the water bath and cook for 2 hours.
3. Once the timer has stopped, remove the medallions and pat them dry. Discard the bay leaf. Reserve cooking juices. Sear in a high hot skillet about 1 minute. Serve with the sauce and mashed potatoes.

Lollipop Lamb Chops

Servings: 4
Cooking Time: 60 Minutes
Ingredients:
- 8 lollipop lamb chops
- 1 tablespoon olive oil
- ½ teaspoon Garam Masala
- ¼ teaspoon lemon pepper
- ½ tablespoon garlic powder
- Salt and pepper as needed
- ½ cup yogurt
- ¼ cup fresh cilantro, chopped
- 2 tablespoons mango chutney
- 1 tablespoon curry powder
- 1 tablespoon onion, finely chopped
- 1 tablespoon oil

Directions:
1. Prepare the Sous Vide water bath using your immersion circulator and increase the temperature to 140-degrees Fahrenheit
2. Lay chops on a cutting board and drizzle with olive oil
3. Sprinkle both sides with garam masala, lemon pepper, garlic powder, salt and pepper.
4. Place the chops in a zip bag and seal using the immersion method. Cook for 1 hour
5. While the lamb is underwater, start preparing the sauce by thoroughly mixing the yogurt, mango chutney, cilantro, curry powder, and onion in a bowl
6. Transfer to small dish
7. Once the chops are ready, remove from the bag and pat dry
8. Take a skillet and heat up 1 tablespoon of oil, over high heat, and add the chops when smoking hot
9. Sear the chops for 30 seconds per side and remove from the skillet. Drain quickly on a kitchen towel
10. Serve the chops by arranging them on a serving platter. Place the yogurt sauce on the side
11. Garnish with some chopped cilantro on top

Nutrition Info: Per serving:Calories: 927 ;Carbohydrate: 3g ;Protein: 35g ;Fat: 85g ;Sugar: 2g ;Sodium: 447mg

Loin Pork With Almonds

Servings: 2
Cooking Time: 3 Hours 20 Minutes
Ingredients:
- 3 tbsp olive oil
- 3 tbsp mustard
- 2 tbsp honey
- Salt and black pepper to taste
- 2 bone-in pork loin chops
- 1 tbsp lemon juice
- 2 tsp red wine vinegar
- 2 tbsp canola oil
- 2 cups mixed baby lettuce
- 2 tbsp thinly sliced sundried tomatoes
- 2 tsp almonds, toasted

Directions:
1. Prepare a water bath and place the Sous Vide in it. Set to 138 F.
2. Combine 1 tbsp of olive oil, 1 tbsp of honey, and 1 tbsp of mustard and season with salt and pepper. Brush the loin with the mixture. Place in a vacuum-sealable bag. Release air by the water displacement method, seal and submerge the bag in the water bath. Cook for 3 hours.
3. Meanwhile, prepare the dressing mixing the lemon juice, vinegar, 2 tbsp of olive oil, 2 tbsp of mustard, and the remaining honey. Season with salt and pepper. Once the timer has stopped, remove the loin. Discard cooking juices. Heat canola oil in a skillet over high heat and sear the loin for 30 seconds per side. Allow resting for 5 minutes.
4. For the salad, combine in a bowl the lettuce, sun-dried tomatoes and almonds. Mix in 3/4 of the dressing Top loin with the dressing and serve with the salad.

FISH & SEAFOOD RECIPES

Swordfish With Mango Salsa

Cooking Time: 35 Mins Cooking Temperature: 127°f

Ingredients:

- For Salsa:
- 5½ ounces fresh raspberries, washed
- 5½ ounces fresh mango, peeled, pitted and chopped
- 1½ ounces red onion, minced
- ⅓ cup fresh cilantro, chopped
- 1 small jalapeño pepper, minced
- 2 tablespoons fresh lime juice
- For Swordfish:
- 3 tablespoons sugar
- 3 tablespoons fine sea salt
- 4-4½ cups cool water
- 4 x 4-ounce swordfish fillets
- ½ cup butter
- 3 tablespoons balsamic vinegar
- 1¾ tablespoons honey
- 1½ tablespoons Dijon mustard
- salt and freshly ground white pepper, to taste

Directions:

1. For the salsa:
2. to a bowl, add all ingredients and mix. Refrigerate overnight, covered.
3. For the swordfish:
4. in a large bowl, dissolve sugar and salt in cool water. Place swordfish fillets and refrigerate for 3 hours.
5. Attach the sous vide immersion circulator using an adjustable clamp to a Cambro container or pot filled with water and preheat to 127°F.
6. Into a pan, add butter and cook until golden brown, swirling pan continuously.
7. Remove from heat and add vinegar, honey, Dijon mustard, salt and white pepper, beating until well-combined.
8. Remove fish fillet from bowl of cold water and lightly season with salt and white pepper.
9. Between 4 cooking pouches, divide fish fillets. Add 2-3 tablespoons of brown butter to each pouch. Seal pouches tightly after squeezing out the excess air.
10. Place pouches in sous vide bath and set the cooking time for 30 minutes.
11. Remove pouches from sous vide bath and carefully open them. Remove fish fillets from pouches. With paper towels, pat fillets completely dry.
12. With a blow torch, toast each fillet until a slight crust is formed.
13. Divide fillets onto serving plates and drizzle evenly with brown butter.
14. Place salsa evenly alongside each fillet and serve.

Chili Smelts

Servings: 5

Cooking Time: 1 Hour 15 Minutes

Ingredients:

- 1 pound fresh smelts
- ½ cup lemon juice
- 3 garlic cloves, crushed
- 1 tsp salt
- 1 cup extra virgin olive oil
- 2 tbsp fresh dill, finely chopped
- 1 tbsp chives, minced
- 1 tbsp chili pepper, ground

Directions:

1. Rinse smelts under cold running water and drain. Set aside.
2. In a large bowl, combine olive oil with lemon juice, crushed garlic, sea salt, finely chopped dill, minced chives, and chili pepper. Place smelts into this mixture and cover. Refrigerate for 20 minutes.
3. Remove from the refrigerator and place in a large vacuum-sealable bag along with the marinade. Cook in sous vide for 40 minutes at 104 F. Remove from the water bath and drain but reserve the liquid.
4. Heat a large skillet over medium heat. Add smelts and briefly cook, for 3-4 minutes, turning them over. Remove from the heat and transfer to a serving plate. Drizzle with marinade and serve immediately.

Smoked Prawn

Servings: 2

Cooking Time: 15 Minutes

Ingredients:

- 24 pieces of de-shelled small prawns
- 4 tablespoons extra-virgin olive oil
- Smoked salt
- Pepper as needed

Directions:

1. Take a large-sized pot of water and heat to a temperature of 149-degrees Fahrenheit using your Sous Vide immersion circulator
2. Add the prawns, olive oil, pepper and smoked salt in a heavy-duty plastic zipper bag
3. Seal it using the immersion method, and cook for 15 minutes
4. Once cooked, place the prawns in a hot pan and sear until they turn golden brown
5. Add some extra smoked salt to enhance the flavors.
6. Serve!

Nutrition Info: Calories: 560 Carbohydrate: 86g Protein: 25g Fat: 12g Sugar: 11g Sodium: 390mg

Pan Tomate Espelette Shrimp

Servings: 4

Cooking Time: 25 Minutes

Ingredients:

- 1 lb. shrimps, peeled, de-veined
- 1 tablespoon extra-virgin olive oil
- ¾ teaspoon Piment d'Espelette
- Kosher salt as needed
- ½ high-quality loaf of bread cut up into 1½ inch slices
- 1 garlic clove, halved
- 2 beefsteak tomatoes, 1 sliced horizontally, the other sliced into wedges
- Flaky sea salt

Directions:

1. Prepare your Sous-vide water bath to a temperature of 122ºF
2. Take a large-sized bowl and put the shrimps in it along with the olive oil, a pinch of kosher salt and the Piment d'Espelette
3. Whisk it well and transfer the mixture to a large-sized heavy-duty zip bag. Seal the bag using the immersion method

4. Submerge the bag underwater and cook for 25 minutes
5. Place a grill pan over a medium-high heat for 5 minutes before the shrimps are done
6. Carefully arrange the bread slices in a single layer in your pan and toast them on both sides
7. Once toasted, remove the bread and rub one side of the slices with the garlic clove
8. Rub the tomato halves over your toast as well and divide them between your serving plates
9. Once cooked, remove the bag and drain the liquid
10. Return the grill pan to a medium-high heat and add the shrimp a single layer
11. Sear for 10 seconds and divide the shrimps among the tomato bread
12. Drizzle the olive oil over your shrimps Sprinkle some salt over and serve with the tomato wedges! **Nutrition Info:** Per serving:Calories 238, Carbohydrates 25 g, Fats 6 g, Protein 21 g

Crab Zucchini Roulade With Mousse

Servings: 4

Cooking Time: 10 Minutes

Ingredients:

- 3lb. crab legs and claws
- 2 tablespoons olive oil
- 1 medium zucchini
- Salt and pepper, to taste
- Mousse:
- 1 avocado, peeled, pitted
- 1 tablespoon Worcestershire sauce
- 2 tablespoons crème Fraiche
- 2 tablespoons fresh lime juice
- Salt, to taste

Directions:

1. Preheat Sous vide cooker to 185F.
2. Place the claws and legs in a Sous Vide bag and vacuum seal.
3. Submerge the bag with content in a water bath. Cook the crab 10 minutes.
4. Finishing steps:
5. Slice the zucchini with a vegetable peeler. This way you will have some skinny strips.

6. Remove the crab from the water bath and crack the shell.

7. Flake the meat and transfer into a bowl. Add olive oil, salt, and pepper, and stir to bind gently.

8. Make the mousse; in a food blender, blend the avocado and crème Fraiche until smooth.

9. Stir in the remaining ingredients and spoon the mixture into piping bag.

10. Arrange the zucchini slices on aluminum foil and fill with the crab meat.

11. Roll up the zucchinis and crab into a log and refrigerate 30 minutes.

12. To serve; cut the roulade into four pieces. Serve onto a plate with some avocado mousse.

13. Enjoy.

Nutrition Info: Calories 415 Total Fat 11g Total Carb 6g Dietary Fiber 5g Protein 43g

Salmon Patties

Servings: 4
Cooking Time: 45 Minutes
Ingredients:

- 1 pound boneless skinless salmon fillets
- 4 tablespoons olive oil /divided
- 2 eggs /lightly beaten
- 1/4 cup chopped parsley
- 1/4 cup Italian-seasoned Panko breadcrumbs
- 2 tablespoons chopped onion
- 1 lemon /zested, juiced
- 2 tablespoons chopped fresh basil leaves
- 1/4 teaspoon red pepper flakes
- Salt and freshly ground black pepper, to taste

Directions:

1. Preheat water to 105°F in a sous vide cooker or with an immersion circulator.

2. Vacuum-seal salmon and 2 tablespoons olive oil in a sous vide bag, or use a plastic zip-top freezer bag /remove as much air as possible from the bag before sealing. Submerge bag in water and cook for 30 minutes.

3. Remove salmon from cooking bag and flake coarsely with a fork. Mix salmon, eggs, parsley, breadcrumbs, onion, lemon juice, basil and red pepper flakes and season to taste with salt and pepper. Stir mixture until thoroughly combined and form into four firmly packed patties.

4. Heat remaining 2 tablespoons oil in a large nonstick skillet over medium heat and fry salmon patties until browned on both sides, about 4 minutes per side. Sprinkle salmon patties with lemon zest and serve immediately. Enjoy!

Nutrition Info: Calories: 356; Total Fat: 22g; Saturated Fat: 4g; Protein: 33g; Carbs: 7g; Fiber: 1g; Sugar: 1g

Red Snapper

Cooking Time: 30 Mins Cooking Temperature: 132°f
Ingredients:

- 30-ounce skinless red snapper fillet, cut into 6 pieces and chilled
- 6 small, fresh bay leaves
- A few strings of freshly cut chilies
- 1 teaspoon fennel seeds
- sea salt, to taste
- 1½ tablespoons cold butter, cubed

Directions:

1. Attach the sous vide immersion circulator using an adjustable clamp to a Cambro container or pot filled with water and preheat to 132°F.

2. Into a large cooking pouch, place snapper pieces, bay leaves, chilies and fennel seeds. Seal pouch tightly after squeezing out the excess air. Place pouch in sous vide bath and set the cooking time for 25 minutes.

3. Remove pouch from sous vide bath and carefully open it. Remove fillets from pouch, reserving cooking liquid.

4. Transfer fillets onto warm serving plates and sprinkle with salt.

5. Into a small pan, add butter and reserved cooking liquid, and cook until desired thickness is achieved.

6. Pour sauce over snapper fillets and serve.

Sweet Mango Shrimp

Servings: 4
Cooking Time: 15 Minutes
Ingredients:

- 24 medium-sized shrimps, peeled and de-veined
- 4 pieces' mangoes, peeled and shredded, cut into thin strips
- 2 medium-sized shallots, thinly-sliced
- ¾ cup halved cherry tomatoes
- 2 tablespoons chopped, fresh Thai basil leaves
- ¼ cup toasted dry pan peanuts
- For Thai Dressing
- ¼ cup freshly squeeze lime juice
- 6 tablespoons palm sugar
- 5 tablespoons fish sauce
- 4-8 pieces' garlic cloves
- 4-8 pieces small red chili

Directions:

1. Prepare your Sous-vide water bath to a temperature of 135-degrees Fahrenheit
2. Take a heavy-duty, large resealable zipper bag and layer the shrimp in a single layer inside
3. Seal the bag using the immersion method. Submerge under water and cook for 15 minutes
4. Put the lime juice, fish sauce, and palm sugar in a small bowl and mix well
5. Take a mortar and pestle and pound well the garlic
6. Add the chilis and keep pounding
7. Whisk well, then add the mixture to the dressing
8. Once the shrimps are ready, take them out
9. Transfer them to a large-sized bowl
10. Add the green mango strips, Thai basil, shallots, tomato halves and peanuts to the bowl
11. Top off with the dressing and serve!

Nutrition Info: Calories: 245 Carbohydrate: 11g Protein: 19g Fat: 11g Sugar: 5g Sodium: 532mg

Coriander-garlic Squids

Servings: 4
Cooking Time: 2 Hours
Ingredients:
- 4 4oz. squids, cleaned
- ¼ cup olive oil
- ¼ cup chopped coriander
- 4 cloves garlic, minced
- 2 chili pepper, chopped
- 2 teaspoons minced ginger
- ¼ cup vegetable oil

- 1 lemon, cut into wedges
- Salt and pepper, to taste

Directions:

1. Set the Sous vide cooker to 136F.
2. Place the squids and 2 tablespoons olive oil in a Sous Vide bags. Season to taste and vacuum seal the bag.
3. Submerge in water and cook 2 hours.
4. Finishing steps:
5. Heat remaining olive oil in a skillet. Add garlic, chili pepper, and ginger and cook 1 minute. Add half the coriander and stir well. Remove from the heat.
6. Remove the squids from the bag.
7. Heat vegetable oil in a skillet, until sizzling hot. Add the squid and cook 30 seconds per side.
8. Transfer the squids onto a plate. Top with garlic-coriander mixture and sprinkle with the remaining coriander.
9. Serve with lemon.

Nutrition Info: Calories 346 Total Fat 29g Total Carb 7g Dietary Fiber 7g Protein 12g

Crispy Skinned Salmon

Servings: 2
Cooking Time: 8 Minutes
Ingredients:
- 2 skin-on salmon fillets
- Salt and black pepper as needed
- 1 tablespoon extra-virgin olive oil
- 4½ tablespoons soy sauce
- 2 tablespoons minced fresh ginger
- 2 thinly sliced Thai Chilis
- 6 tablespoons sesame oil
- 4 ounces prepared Chinese egg noodles
- 6 oz. cooked broccolini
- 5 teaspoons sesame seeds for garnishing, toasted

Directions:

1. Prepare your Sous-vide water bath to a temperature of 149-degrees Fahrenheit
2. Skin the salmon and transfer them to a parchment paper-lined baking sheet. Season with salt and pepper
3. Take a sheet and lay it on top of the skin and place another baking sheet on top

4. Transfer to an oven and bake for 30 minutes
5. Season with salt and pepper and transfer the baked salmon to large-sized, resealable zipper bag
6. Seal the bag using the immersion method, submerge underwater and cook for 8 minutes
7. Take a small-sized bowl and add the ginger, chilis, 4 tablespoons of soy sauce, 4 tablespoons of sesame oil and whisk everything well to prepare the dipping sauce
8. Divide it all between two serving bowls
9. Toss the noodles and broccolini with 2 teaspoons of sesame oil and ½ teaspoon of soy sauce
10. Divide it between two serving plates as well
11. Once cooked, remove the contents of the bag and place one fillet on the bed of noodles
12. Garnish with some toasted sesame seeds and salmon skin
13. Serve the salmon alongside the sauce

Nutrition Info: Calories: 649 Carbohydrate: 117g Protein: 31g Fat: 6g Sugar: 0g Sodium: 492mg

Seared Tuna Steaks

Servings: 4
Cooking Time: 40 Minutes
Ingredients:

- 2 tuna steaks /1" thick, about 10 ounces each
- 1 teaspoon kosher salt
- 1/4 teaspoon cayenne pepper
- 3 tablespoons olive oil /divided
- 1 teaspoon butter
- 1 tablespoon whole peppercorns

Directions:
1. Preheat water to 105°F in a sous vide cooker or with an immersion circulator.
2. Season tuna steaks with salt and cayenne pepper and vacuum-seal with 1 tablespoon olive oil in a sous vide bag, or use a plastic zip-top freezer bag /remove as much air as possible from the bag before sealing. Submerge bag in water and cook for 30 minutes.
3. Remove tuna steaks from bag and blot dry with paper towels. Heat remaining 2 tablespoons olive oil and butter in a large nonstick skillet over medium-high heat. Cook peppercorns until softened and beginning to pop, about 5 minutes. Place tuna steaks

in skillet and sear until browned, about 1 minute per side. Cut tuna steaks in half and serve with the peppercorns from the skillet. Enjoy!

Nutrition Info: Calories: 359; Total Fat: 20g; Saturated Fat: 4g; Protein: 42g; Carbs: 0g; Fiber: 0g; Sugar: 0g

Dublin-style Lemon Shrimp Dish

Servings: 4
Cooking Time: 1 Hour 15 Minutes
Ingredients:

- 4 tbsp butter
- 2 tbsp lime juice
- 2 cloves fresh garlic, minced
- 1 tsp fresh lime zest
- Salt and black pepper to taste
- 1 pound jumbo shrimp, peeled and de-veined
- ½ cup of panko bread crumbs
- 1 tbsp fresh parsley, minced

Directions:
1. Prepare a water bath and place the Sous Vide in it. Set to 135 F.
2. Heat 3 tbsp of butter in a skillet over medium heat and add in lime juice, salt, pepper, garlic, and zest. Allow cooling for 5 minutes. Place the shrimp and mixture in a vacuum-sealable bag. Release air by the water displacement method, seal and submerge the bag in the water bath. Cook for 30 minutes.
3. Meanwhile, heat butter in a pan over medium and toast the panko breadcrumbs. Once the timer has stopped, remove the shrimp and transfer to a hot pot over high heat and cook with the cooking juices. Serve in 4 soup bowls and top with the breadcrumbs.

Buttery Red Snapper With Citrus Saffron Sauce

Servings: 4
Cooking Time: 55 Minutes
Ingredients:

- 4 pieces cleaned red snapper
- 2 tbsp butter
- Salt and black pepper to taste
- For Citrus Sauce
- 1 lemon

- 1 grapefruit
- 1 lime
- 3 oranges
- 1 tsp Dijon mustard
- 2 tbsp canola oil
- 1 yellow onion
- 1 diced zucchini
- 1 tsp saffron threads
- 1 tsp diced chili pepper
- 1 tbsp sugar
- 3 cups fish stock
- 3 tbsp chopped cilantro

Directions:

1. Prepare a water bath and place the Sous Vide in it. Set to 132 F. Season the snapper fillets with salt and pepper and place in a vacuum-sealable bag. Release air by the water displacement method, seal and submerge the bag in the water bath. Cook for 30 minutes.
2. Peel the fruits and chop in cubes. Heat oil in a skillet over medium heat and put the onion and zucchini. Sauté for 2-3 minutes. Add the fruits, saffron, pepper, mustard and sugar. Cook for 1 minute more. Stir the fish stock and simmer for 10 minutes. Garnish with cilantro, and set aside. Once the timer has stopped, remove the fish and transfer to a plate. Glaze with citrus-saffron sauce and serve.

Perfect Scallops In Citrus Sauce

Servings: 4
Cooking Time: 30 Minutes
Ingredients:

- 2lb. scallops, cleaned
- 2 lemons /1 quartered, 1 zested and juiced
- 2 tablespoons ghee
- 2 shallots, chopped
- ¼ cup pink grapefruit juice
- ¼ cup orange juice
- 2 tablespoons acacia honey
- Salt and pepper, to taste

Directions:

1. Preheat Souse Vide cooker to 122F.
2. Rinse scallops and drain.
3. Season scallops with salt and pepper. Divide scallops between two Sous Vide bags.

4. Place 2 quarters lemon in each bag and vacuum seal.
5. Cook the scallops 30 minutes.
6. Finishing steps:
7. Make the sauce; heat ghee in a saucepan.
8. Add the chopped shallots and cook until tender 4 minutes.
9. Remove the scallops from the bag and sear on both sides in a lightly greased skillet.
10. Remove the scallops from the skillet.
11. Deglaze the pan with orange juice. Pour in pink grapefruit juice and lemon juice.
12. Add shallots and lemon zest. Simmer until half reduces the sauce. Stir in honey and simmer until thickened.
13. Serve scallops with sauce.

Nutrition Info: Calories 279 Total Fat 2g Total Carb 17g Dietary Fiber 1g Protein 37g

Shrimp With Creamy Wine Sauce

Servings: 4
Cooking Time: 30 Minutes
Ingredients:

- 1 pound large shrimp /peeled, deveined
- 2 garlic cloves /sliced
- 1/4 teaspoon salt
- 1/4 teaspoon freshly ground black pepper
- 1 tablespoon olive oil
- 2 shallots /minced
- 3/4 cup white wine
- 2 tablespoons butter /softened
- 2 tablespoons cream cheese /softened
- 2 tablespoons chopped fresh parsley leaves
- 1 tablespoon freshly grated Parmesan cheese
- 1 teaspoon red pepper flakes

Directions:

1. Preheat water to 140°F in a sous vide cooker or with an immersion circulator.
2. Vacuum-seal shrimp, garlic, salt and pepper in a sous vide bag, or use a plastic zip-top freezer bag /remove as much air as possible from the bag before sealing. Arrange shrimp in a single layer in bag, submerge bag in water and cook for 30 minutes.
3. Meanwhile, for the sauce, heat olive oil in a large nonstick skillet over medium heat and sauté shallots

for about 3 minutes. Add wine and simmer to reduce, stirring occasionally, 3-4 minutes. Add butter and cream cheese to sauce and whisk until melted and incorporated.

4.   Pour shrimp into sauce and stir to coat. Transfer shrimp and sauce to a bowl and sprinkle with parsley, Parmesan cheese and red pepper flakes to serve. Enjoy!

Nutrition Info: Calories: 257; Total Fat: 12g; Saturated Fat: 6g; Protein: 24g; Carbs: 6g; Fiber: 0g; Sugar: 1g

Fish Tacos

Cooking Time: 20 Mins Cooking Temperature: 132°f
Ingredients:
- For Fish:
- 1 teaspoons fresh cilantro, chopped
- ½ teaspoon chili powder
- pinch of salt and freshly ground black pepper
- 1 pound thick, flaky fish (cod/halibut)
- For Marinated Onion:
- ½ large red onion, thinly sliced
- 1 tablespoon white wine vinegar
- 1 teaspoons fresh cilantro, chopped
- pinch of salt and freshly ground black pepper
- For Tacos:
- ⅓ cup sour cream
- 1 teaspoon hot sauce
- 4 corn or flour tortillas
- lettuce, as required, shredded
- 1 avocado, peeled, pitted and sliced
- 10-12 cherry tomatoes, halved
- 4 lime wedges

Directions:
1.   Attach the sous vide immersion circulator using an adjustable clamp to a Cambro container or pot filled with water and preheat to 132°F.
2.   For the fish:
3.   in a small bowl, mix together cilantro, chili powder, salt and black pepper. Season fish with cilantro mixture evenly.
4.   Into a cooking pouch, add fish. Seal pouch tightly after squeezing out the excess air. Place pouch in sous vide bath and set the cooking time for 20 minutes.

5.   Meanwhile for the marinated onion:
6.   in a small bowl, mix together all ingredients and keep aside.
7.   In another bowl, mix together sour cream and hot sauce and keep aside.
8.   Remove pouch from sous vide bath and carefully open it. Remove fish from pouch.
9.   Arrange tacos onto serving plates.
10.   Place a heaped spoonful of cooked fish onto the center of each tortilla. Top with the shredded lettuce, followed by marinated onion, avocado and tomato evenly.
11.   Drizzle with sour cream and serve alongside lime wedges.

Buttery Cockles With Peppercorns

Servings: 2
Cooking Time: 1 Hour 30 Minutes
Ingredients:
- 4 oz canned cockles
- ¼ cup dry white wine
- 1 diced celery stalk
- 1 diced parsnip
- 1 quartered shallot
- 1 bay leaf
- 1 tbsp black peppercorns
- 1 tbsp olive oil
- 8 tbsp butter, room temperature
- 1 tbsp minced fresh parsley
- 2 garlic cloves, minced
- Salt to taste
- 1 tsp freshly cracked black pepper
- ¼ cup panko breadcrumbs
- 1 baguette, sliced

Directions:
1.   Prepare a water bath and place the Sous Vide in it. Set to 154 F. Place the cockles, shallots, celery, parsnip, wine, peppercorns, olive oil and bay leaf in a vacuum-sealable bag. Release air by the water displacement method, seal and submerge the bag in the water bath. Cook for 60 minutes.
2.   Using a blender, pour the butter, parsley, salt, garlic and ground pepper. Mix at medium speed until combined. Put the mixture into a plastic bag and roll it. Move into the fridge and allow chilling.

3. Once the timer has stopped, remove the snail and veggies. Discard the cooking juices. Heat a skillet over high heat. Top the cockles with butter, sprinkle some breadcrumbs over and cook for 3 minutes until melted. Serve with warm baguette slices.

Shrimps Cajun

Servings: 4
Cooking Time: 25 Minutes
Ingredients:
- 16 shrimps, peeled and deveined
- 1 shallot, minced
- 1 tbsp unsalted butter, melted
- 1 tbsp Cajun seasoning
- 2 garlic cloves, minced
- 1 tbsp lemon juice
- Freshly ground black pepper to taste
- 4 tbsp freshly chopped parsley

Directions:
1. Preheat your cooking machine to 125ºF.
2. Put all ingredients except parsley into the vacuum bag.
3. Seal the bag, put it into the water bath and set the timer for 25 minutes.
4. Serve immediately as an appetizer garnished with the chopped parsley.

Nutrition Info: Per serving:Calories 167, Carbohydrates 8 g, Fats 7 g, Protein 18 g

Coconut Cod Stew

Servings: 6
Cooking Time: 30 Minutes
Ingredients:
- 2 pounds fresh cod /cut into fillets
- Salt and freshly ground black pepper, to taste
- 1 can /15 ounces coconut milk /divided
- 1 tablespoon olive oil
- 1 sweet onion /julienned
- 1 red bell pepper /julienned
- 4 garlic cloves /minced
- 1 can /15 ounces crushed tomatoes
- 1 teaspoon fish sauce
- 1 teaspoon lime juice

- Sriracha hot sauce, to taste
- 2 tablespoon chopped fresh cilantro leaves

Directions:
1. Preheat water to 130°F in a sous vide cooker or with an immersion circulator.
2. Season cod fillets with salt and pepper and vacuum-seal with 1/4 cup coconut milk in a sous vide bag /or use a plastic zip-top freezer bag, removing as much air as possible from the bag before sealing. Submerge bag in water and cook for 30 minutes.
3. Immediately begin preparing the sauce. Heat olive oil in a nonstick skillet over medium-high heat and sauté onion and bell pepper until softened, 3 to 4 minutes, stirring frequently. Add garlic and sauté about 1 minute more, stirring constantly. Add undrained tomatoes, fish sauce, lime juice, sriracha sauce and remaining coconut milk and stir until thoroughly combined. Season sauce to taste with salt and pepper, reduce heat to low and simmer until the end of the cooking time for the cod, stirring occasionally.
4. Remove cod from cooking bag, add to sauce and turn gently to coat with sauce. Let stew stand for about 5 minutes. Garnish stew with cilantro leaves to serve. Enjoy!

Nutrition Info: Calories: 400; Total Fat: 18g; Saturated Fat: 13g; Protein: 40g; Carbs: 23g; Fiber: 5g; Sugar: 2g

Sous Vide Lobster Rolls

Servings: 2
Cooking Time: 45 Minutes
Ingredients:
- 2 lobster tails, cut into ½ inch pieces
- 6 tablespoons unsalted butter
- 1 teaspoon sea salt
- 1 teaspoon chopped, fresh tarragon
- 1 teaspoon chopped chives
- ½ teaspoon garlic powder
- 1 teaspoon lemon zest
- 2 toasted hot dog buns for serving

Directions:
1. Prepare your Sous-vide water bath to a temperature of 122-degrees Fahrenheit

2. Add the salt, butter, lobster, garlic powder, tarragon, lemon zest, and chives in a heavy-duty, resealable zip bag and seal using the immersion method
3. Submerge and cook for 45 minutes
4. Once done, remove from the water bath and put the lobsters in a medium sized bowl
5. Pour in some of extra butter
6. Place the lobster pieces in the hot dog buns and serve with extra butter

Nutrition Info: Calories: 348 Carbohydrate: 7g Protein: 24g Fat: 2g Sugar: 3g Sodium: 358mg

Divine Garlic-lemon Crab Rolls

Servings: 4
Cooking Time: 60 Minutes
Ingredients:
- 4 tbsp butter
- 1 pound cooked crabmeat
- 2 garlic cloves, minced
- Zest and juice of ½ lemon
- ½ cup mayonnaise
- 1 fennel bulb, chopped
- Salt and black pepper to taste
- 4 rolls, split, oiled, and toasted

Directions:
1. Prepare a water bath and place Sous Vide in it. Set to 137 F. Combine garlic, lemon zest and 1/4 cup of lemon juice. Place the crabmeat in a vacuum-sealable bag with butter and lemon mix. Release air by the water displacement method, seal and submerge the bag in the water bath. Cook for 50 minutes.
2. Once the timer has stopped, remove the bag and transfer into a bowl. Discard the cooking juices. Combine the crabmeat with the remaining lemon juice, mayonnaise, fennel, dill, salt, and pepper. Fill the rolls with the crabmeat mixture before serving.

Lazy Man's Lobster

Servings: 1
Cooking Time: 1 Hr.
Ingredients:
- Tail and claws of 1 lobster

- 2 tablespoons butter
- 1 clove garlic, minced
- ½ tablespoon fresh thyme, minced
- ¼ cup sherry
- ½ teaspoon salt
- ½ teaspoon pepper
- ¼ cup heavy cream
- Toast for serving

Directions:
1. Preheat the water bath to 140°F. Seal lobster into the bag. Place in water bath and cook 1 hour. Meanwhile, prepare the sauce. Melt butter in a pan. Add garlic and thyme and cook 30 seconds. Add sherry and bring to a boil. Remove from heat and stir in cream. Season with salt and pepper. When lobster is cooked, remove the shell and stir into sauce. Serve with toast.

Nutrition Info: Calories: 582 Protein: 27gCarbs: 45gFat: 426g

Curry Mackerel

Servings: 3
Cooking Time: 55 Minutes
Ingredients:
- 3 mackerel filets, heads removed
- 3 tbsp curry paste
- 1 tbsp olive oil
- Salt and black pepper to taste

Directions:
1. Make a water bath, place Sous Vide in it, and set to 120 F. Season the mackerel with pepper and salt and place in a vacuum-sealable bag. Release air by the water displacement method, seal and submerge it in the water bath, and set the timer for 40 minutes.
2. Once the timer has stopped, remove and unseal the bag. Set a skillet over medium heat, add olive oil. Coat the mackerel with the curry powder (do not pat the mackerel dry)
3. Once it has heated, add the mackerel and sear until golden brown. Serve with a side of steamed green leafy vegetables.

Tasty Trout With Mustard & Tamari Sauce

Servings: 4

Cooking Time: 35 Minutes

Ingredients:

- ¼ cup olive oil
- 4 trout fillets, skinned and sliced
- ½ cup Tamari sauce
- ¼ cup light brown sugar
- 2 garlic cloves, minced
- 1 tbsp Coleman's mustard

Directions:

1. Prepare a water bath and place Sous Vide in it. Set to 130 F. Combine the Tamari sauce, brown sugar, olive oil, and garlic. Place the trout in a vacuum-sealable bag with tamari mixture. Release air by the water displacement method, seal and submerge the bag in the water bath. Cook for 30 minutes.
2. Once the timer has stopped, remove the trout and pat dry with kitchen towel. Discard the cooking juices. Garnish with tamari sauce and mustard to serve.

Baby Octopus Dish

Servings: 4
Cooking Time: 50 Minutes

Ingredients:

- 1 lb. baby octopus
- 1 tablespoon extra-virgin olive oil
- 1 tablespoon lemon juice, freshly squeezed
- Kosher salt and black pepper as needed

Directions:

1. Prepare your Sous-vide water bath to a temperature of 134-degrees Fahrenheit
2. Add the octopus in a heavy-duty resealable zipper bag
3. Seal the bag using the immersion method and cook underwater for 50 minutes
4. Once cooked, remove the octopus and pat it dry
5. Toss the cooked octopus with some olive oil and lemon juice and season it with salt and pepper
6. Serve!

Nutrition Info: Calories: 378 Carbohydrate: 4g Protein: 25g Fat: 29g Sugar: 0g Sodium: 392mg Special Tips If you want a nice crispy chard, grill the cooked and seasoned octopus for 1 minute on each side.

Cilantro Trout

Servings: 4
Cooking Time: 60 Minutes

Ingredients:

- 2 pounds trout, 4 pieces
- 5 garlic cloves
- 1 tbsp sea salt
- 4 tbsp olive oil
- 1 cup cilantro leaves, finely chopped
- 2 tbsp rosemary, finely chopped
- ¼ cup freshly squeezed lemon juice

Directions:

1. Clean and rinse well the fish. Pat dry with a kitchen paper and rub with salt. Combine garlic with olive oil, cilantro, rosemary, and lemon juice. Use the mixture to fill each fish. Place in a separate vacuum-sealable bags and seal. Cook en Sous Vide for 45 minutes at 131 F.

Mussels In Fresh Lime Juice

Servings: 2
Cooking Time: 40 Minutes

Ingredients:

- 1 pound fresh mussels, debearded
- 1 medium-sized onion, peeled and finely chopped
- Garlic cloves, crushed
- ½ cup freshly squeezed lime juice
- ¼ cup fresh parsley, finely chopped
- 1 tbsp rosemary, finely chopped
- 2 tbsp olive oil

Directions:

1. Place mussels along with lime juice, garlic, onion, parsley, rosemary, and olive oil in a large vacuum-sealable bag. Cook en Sous Vide for 30 minutes at 122 F. Serve with green salad.

Black Cod

Cooking Time: 35 Mins Cooking Temperature: 130°f

Ingredients:

- 2 medium bone-in black cod fillets
- 1 x 1-inch piece fresh ginger, grated
- 1 cup soy sauce

- ½ cup mirin
- 2 dashes fish sauce

Directions:

1. Attach the sous vide immersion circulator using an adjustable clamp to a Cambro container or pot filled with water and preheat to 130°F.
2. Into a cooking pouch, add all ingredients. Seal pouch tightly after squeezing out the excess air. Place pouch in sous vide bath and set the cooking time for 30 minutes.
3. Preheat broiler to high.
4. Remove pouch from sous vide bath and carefully open it. Remove fillets from pouch. With paper towels, pat fillets completely dry.
5. Broil until golden brown.

Salmon Egg Bites

Servings: 6
Cooking Time: 60 Minutes
Ingredients:
- 6 whole eggs
- ¼ cup crème fraiche
- ¼ cup cream cheese
- 4 spears asparagus
- 2 oz. smoked salmon
- 2 oz. chèvre
- ½ oz. minced shallot
- 2 teaspoons chopped, fresh dill
- Salt and pepper as needed
- Tools Required:
- 6 x 4 oz. canning jars

Directions:

1. Prepare your Sous-vide water bath to a temperature of 170-degrees Fahrenheit
2. Add the eggs, cream fraiche, cream cheese and salt into a blender
3. Chop the asparagus into ½ cm chunks. Add them in a mixing bowl with the shallots
4. Chop the salmon into small portions and add them to your shallots
5. Whisk well with some minced dill
6. Whisk everything with a fork
7. Lay out the canning jars and add the egg mixture between them

8. Divide the salmon mix into six and put one portion in each jar
9. Add 1/6 chèvre into the jars and lock the lid to fingertip tightness
10. Put them into the water bath and cook for 1 hour
11. Once done, take out from the water bath.
12. Sprinkle some salt over and serve

Nutrition Info: Calories: 589 Carbohydrate: 61g Protein: 28g Fat: 26g Sugar: 9g Sodium: 590mg

Chili Shrimp & Avocado Salad

Servings: 4
Cooking Time: 45 Minutes
Ingredients:
- 1 chopped red onion
- Juice of 2 limes
- 1 tsp olive oil
- ¼ tsp sea salt
- ⅛ tsp white pepper
- 1 pound raw shrimp, peeled and deveined
- 1 diced tomato
- 1 diced avocado
- 1 green chili pepper, seeded and diced
- 1 tbsp chopped cilantro

Directions:

1. Prepare a water bath and place the Sous Vide in it. Set to 148 F.
2. Place the lime juice, red onion, sea salt, white pepper, olive oil, and shrimp in a vacuum-sealable bag. Release air by the water displacement method, seal and submerge the bag in the water bath. Cook for 24 minutes.
3. Once the timer has stopped, remove the bag and transfer to an ice-water bath for 10 minutes. In a bowl, combine the tomato, avocado, green chili pepper, and cilantro. Pour the bag contents on top.

Spiced Charred Octopus With Lemon Sauce

Servings: 4
Cooking Time: 4 Hours 15 Minutes
Ingredients:
- 5 tbsp olive oil

- 1 pound octopus tentacles
- Salt and black pepper to taste
- 2 tbsp lemon juice
- 1 tbsp lemon zest
- 1 tbsp minced fresh parsley
- 1 tsp thyme
- 1 tbsp paprika

Directions:

1. Prepare a water bath and place the Sous Vide in it. Set to 179 F. Cut the tentacles into medium-size lengths. Season with salt and pepper. Place the lengths with olive oil in a vacuum-sealable bag. Release air by the water displacement method, seal and submerge the bag in the water bath. Cook for 4 hours.
2. Once the timer has stopped, remove the octopus and pat pat dry with kitchen towel. Discard the cooking juices. Sprinkle with olive oil.
3. Heat a grill over medium heat and sear the tentacles for 10-15 seconds per side. Set aside. Combine well the lemon juice, lemon zest, paprika, thyme and parsley. Top the octopus with lemon dressing.

Salmon With Lemon Miso Sauce

Cooking Time: 1 Hour Cooking Temperature: 118°f

Ingredients:

- 2 x 4-6-ounce fresh salmon fillets
- 2 tablespoons lemon juice
- 2 tablespoons white miso paste
- salt and freshly ground black pepper, to taste

Directions:

1. Attach the sous vide immersion circulator using an adjustable clamp to a Cambro container or pot filled with water and preheat to 118°F.
2. Into a large cooking pouch, place salmon fillets. Seal pouch tightly after squeezing out the excess air. Place pouch in sous vide bath and set the cooking time for 1 hour.
3. For the sauce:
4. in a bowl, mix together remaining ingredients.
5. Remove pouch from sous vide bath and carefully open it.
6. Transfer salmon fillets onto a serving plate. Top with sauce and serve.

Sesame Tuna With Ginger Sauce

Servings: 6
Cooking Time: 45 Minutes
Ingredients:

- Tuna:
- 3 tuna steaks
- Salt and black pepper to taste
- ⅓ cup olive oil
- 2 tbsp canola oil
- ½ cup black sesame seeds
- ½ cup white sesame seeds
- Ginger Sauce:
- 1 inch ginger, grated
- 2 shallots, minced
- 1 red chili, minced
- 3 tbsp water
- 2 ½ lime juice
- 1 ½ tbsp rice vinegar
- 2 ½ tbsp soy sauce
- 1 tbsp fish sauce
- 1 ½ tbsp sugar
- 1 bunch green lettuce leaves

Directions:

1. Start with the sauce: place a small pan over low heat and add olive oil. Once it has heated, add ginger and chili. Cook for 3 minutes Add sugar and vinegar, stir and cook until sugar dissolves. Add water and bring to a boil. Add in soy sauce, fish sauce, and lime juice and cook for 2 minutes. Set aside to cool.
2. Make a water bath, place Sous Vide in it, and set to 110 F. Season the tuna with salt and pepper and place in 3 separate vacuum-sealable bag. Add olive oil, release air from the bag by the water displacement method, seal and submerge the bag in the water bath. Set the timer for 30 minutes.
3. Once the timer has stopped, remove and unseal the bag. Place tuna aside. Place a skillet over low heat and add canola oil. While heating, mix sesame seeds in a bowl. Pat dry tuna, coat them in sesame seeds and sear top and bottom in heated oil until seeds start to toast.
4. Slice tuna into thin strips. Layer a serving platter with lettuce and arrange tuna on the bed of lettuce. Serve with ginger sauce as a starter.

Prawns Diablo

Cooking Time: 20 Mins Cooking Temperature: 135°f

Ingredients:

- 1½ pound fresh tiger prawns
- 2 tablespoons butter
- 1 tablespoon garlic, minced
- 1 tablespoon fresh cilantro, chopped
- 4 lime wedges
- 1 teaspoon sesame oil
- 1 teaspoon ground coriander
- 1 teaspoon ground cumin
- 1 teaspoon cayenne pepper
- 1 teaspoon chili flakes
- 1 teaspoon kosher salt

Directions:

1. Attach the sous vide immersion circulator using an adjustable clamp to a Cambro container or pot filled with water and preheat to 135°F.
2. Into a cooking pouch, add all ingredients. Seal pouch tightly after squeezing out the excess air. Place pouch in sous vide bath and set the cooking time for 20 minutes.
3. Remove pouch from sous vide bath and carefully open it. Remove prawns from pouch.
4. Serve alongside your favorite salad.

Easy Tilapia

Servings: 3

Cooking Time: 1 Hour 10 Minutes

Ingredients:

- 3 (4 oz) tilapia filets
- 3 tbsp butter
- 1 tbsp apple cider vinegar
- Salt and black pepper to taste

Directions:

1. Make a water bath, place Sous Vide in it, and set to 124 F. Season the tilapia with pepper and salt and place in a vacuum-sealable bag. Release air by the water displacement method and seal the bag. Submerge it in the water bath and set the timer for 1 hour.
2. Once the timer has stopped, remove and unseal the bag. Put a skillet over medium heat and add butter and vinegar. Simmer and stir continually to reduce vinegar by half. Add the tilapia and sear slightly. Season with salt and pepper as desired. Serve with a side of buttered vegetables.

Lobster Rolls

Servings: 2

Cooking Time: 25 Minutes

Ingredients:

- 2 lobster tails
- 1 tablespoon butter
- 2 green onions, chopped
- 3 tablespoons mayonnaise
- A pinch of salt
- A pinch of black pepper
- 2 teaspoons lemon juice
- Buttered Buns for serving

Directions:

1. Prepare your Sous-vide water bath to a temperature of 140-degrees Fahrenheit
2. Pour the water into a small pot and bring to a boil
3. Cut the lobster tails down the center from the top of the shell
4. Once the water has reached boiling point, submerge the lobsters and cook for 90 seconds
5. Remove them and soak in cold water for 5 minutes
6. Crack the shells and remove the tails from the shell
7. Add the shells in a bag and add the butter. Seal the bag using the immersion method, and cook for 25 minutes
8. Remove the tails from the water bath and pat them dry. Place them in a small bowl and chill for 30 minutes
9. Chop up the tail and mix with the mayonnaise, green onions, salt, pepper, and lime juice.
10. Serve with some toasted, buttered buns

Nutrition Info: Per serving:Calories: 556 ;Carbohydrate: 23g ;Protein: 79g ;Fat: 21g ;Sugar: 3g ;Sodium: 513mg

Crab Mango Salad

Servings: 2
Cooking Time: 45 Minutes
Ingredients:
- 2 blue swimmer crabs
- 1 large-sized mango
- ¼ cup halved cherry tomatoes
- 1 cup rocket lettuce
- ¼ julienned red onion
- Salt and pepper as needed
- 2 tablespoons olive oil
- 1 tablespoon lime juice
- 1 tablespoon freshly squeezed orange juice
- 2 teaspoons honey

Directions:
1. Prepare your Sous-vide water bath to a temperature of 154-degrees Fahrenheit
2. Take a pot of water and let it boil
3. Add the crabs in and let them boil for 60 seconds
4. Chop the legs of the crabs, using pincers, and put them in a heavy-duty, resealable bag. Zip it up using the immersion method
5. Submerge underwater and cook for 45 minutes
6. Add the cooked crabs to an ice bath
7. Add all the dressing ingredients in a bowl. Mix them well
8. Take the crab meat out of the crab and transfer to your serving dish
9. Add the dressing to the crab meat and toss well to coat them
10. Serve!

Nutrition Info: Calories: 148 Carbohydrate: 7g
Protein: 24g Fat: 2g Sugar: 3g Sodium: 518mg

Seafood Mix With Tomato, Wine And Parsley

Servings: 4
Cooking Time: 2 Hours
Ingredients:
- 2 pounds seafood mix, thawed
- 1 cup tomatoes in own juice, diced
- ½ cup dry white wine
- 1 bay leaf
- 1 tsp dried oregano
- 2 garlic cloves, minced
- 2 tbsp olive oil
- Salt and pepper to taste
- Lemon juice for sprinkling
- Chopped parsley for sprinkling

Directions:
1. Preheat your cooking machine to 140ºF.
2. Sprinkle the thawed seafood mix with salt and pepper and put it into the vacuum bag adding tomatoes, bay leaf, dried oregano, garlic, olive oil and white wine.
3. Seal the bag, put it into the water bath and cook for 2 hours.
4. Serve over rice sprinkled with freshly chopped parsley and lemon juice.

Nutrition Info: Per serving:Calories 369, Carbohydrates 18 g, Fats 25 g, Protein 18 g

Herby Lemon Salmon

Servings: 2
Cooking Time: 45 Minutes
Ingredients:
- 2 skinless salmon fillets
- Salt and black pepper to taste
- ¾ cup extra virgin olive oil
- 1 shallot, sliced into thin rings
- 1 tbsp basil leaves, lightly chopped
- 1 tsp allspice
- 3 oz mixed greens
- 1 lemon

Directions:
1. Prepare a water bath and place the Sous Vide in it. Set to 128 F.
2. Place the salmon and season with salt and pepper in a vacuum-sealable bag. Add in shallot rings, olive oil, allspice, and basil. Release air by the water displacement method, seal and submerge the bag in the water bath. Cook for 25 minutes.
3. Once the timer has stopped, remove the bag and transfer the salmon to a plate. Mix the cooking juices with some lemon juice and top salmon fillets. Serve.

Spicy Fish Tortillas

Servings: 6

Cooking Time: 35 Minutes

Ingredients:

- ⅓ cup whipping cream
- 4 halibut fillets, skinned
- 1 tsp chopped fresh cilantro
- ¼ tsp red pepper flakes
- Salt and black pepper to taste
- 1 tbsp cider vinegar
- ½ sweet onion, chopped
- 6 tortillas
- Shredded iceberg lettuce
- 1 large tomato, sliced
- Guacamole for garnish
- 1 lime, quartered

Directions:

1. Prepare a water bath and place the Sous Vide in it. Set to 134 F.
2. Combine fillets with the cilantro, red pepper flakes, salt, and pepper. Place in a vacuum-sealable bag. Release air by the water displacement method, submerge the bag in the bath. Cook for 25 minutes.
3. Meantime, mix the cider vinegar, onion, salt, and pepper. Set aside. Once the timer has stopped, remove the fillets and pat dry with kitchen towel. Using a blowtorch and sear the fillets. Chop into chunks. Put the fish over the tortilla, add lettuce, tomato, cream, onion mixture and guacamole. Garnish with lime.

Salted Salmon In Hollandaise Sauce

Servings: 4

Cooking Time: 1 Hour 50 Minutes

Ingredients:

- 4 salmon fillets
- Salt to taste
- Hollandaise Sauce
- 4 tbsp butter
- 1 egg yolk
- 1 tsp lemon juice
- 1 tsp water
- ½ diced shallot
- A pinch of paprika

Directions:

1. Season the salmon with salt. Allow chilling for 30 minutes. Prepare a water bath and place the Sous

Vide in it. Set to 148 F. Place all the sauce ingredients in a vacuum-sealable bag. Release air by the water displacement method, seal and submerge the bag in the water bath. Cook for 45 minutes.

2. Once the timer has stopped, remove the bag. Set aside. Lower the temperature of the Sous Vide to 120 F and place salmon in a vacuum-sealable bag. Release air by the water displacement method, seal and submerge the bag in the water bath. Cook for 30 minutes. Transfer the sauce to a blender and mix until light yellow. Once the timer has stopped, remove the salmon and pat dry. Serve topped with the sauce.

Sous Vide Lobster With Tarragon

Servings: 4

Cooking Time: 1 Hour

Ingredients:

- 1lb. lobster tail, cleaned
- ¾ cup butter, cubed
- 2 sprigs tarragon
- 1 lime, cut into wedges
- Salt, to taste

Directions:

1. Preheat Sous Vide cooker to 134F.
2. In a Sous Vide bag, combine lobster tail, cubed butter, tarragon, and salt.
3. Vacuum seal the bag.
4. Submerge the bag in a water bath and cook 1 hour.
5. Finishing steps:
6. Remove the bag from the water bath.
7. Open carefully, and transfer the lobster onto a plate.
8. Drizzle the lobster tail with cooking/butter sauce.
9. Serve with lime wedges.

Nutrition Info: Calories 412 Total Fat 35g Total Carb 2g Dietary Fiber 5g Protein 21g

Minty Sardines

Servings: 3

Cooking Time: 1 Hour 20 Minutes

Ingredients:

- 2 pounds sardines
- ¼ cup olive oil
- 3 garlic cloves, crushed
- 1 large lemon, freshly juiced
- 2 sprigs fresh mint
- Salt and black pepper to taste

Directions:

1. Wash and clean each fish but keep the skin. Pat dry using a kitchen paper.
2. In a large bowl, combine olive oil with garlic, lemon juice, fresh mint, salt, and pepper. Place the sardines in a large vacuum-sealable bag along with the marinade. Cook in a water bath for one hour at 104 F. Remove from the bath and drain but reserve the sauce. Drizzle fish with sauce and steamed leek.

Blue Cheese Lobster Tails

Servings: 4

Cooking Time: 1 Hour

Ingredients:

- 4 lobster tails, shells removed
- 10 tbsp butter
- Salt and pepper to taste
- Sous Vide Blue Cheese sauce for serving

Directions:

1. Preheat your cooking machine to 135ºF.
2. Sprinkle the lobster tails with salt and pepper.
3. Put the tails into the vacuum bag and add the butter.
4. Seal the bag and set the timer for 1 hour.
5. Drizzle the cooked lobster tails with the cooking liquid and serve with Sous Vide Blue Cheese sauce.

Nutrition Info: Per serving:Calories 240, Carbohydrates 10 g, Fats 12 g, Protein 23 g

Delicious Artichokes With Simple Dip

Servings: 6
Cooking Time: 1 Hour
Ingredients:
- 6 artichokes, trimmed and cut into halves
- 1 ½ sticks butter, room temperature
- 6 cloves garlic, peeled
- 2 teaspoons lemon zest
- Sea salt and freshly ground black pepper, to taste
- 1/2 cup sour cream
- 1/2 cup mayonnaise

Directions:
1. Preheat a sous vide water bath to 183 degrees F.
2. Place trimmed artichokes along with butter, garlic, lemon zest, salt and black pepper in cooking pouches; seal tightly.
3. Submerge the cooking pouches in the water bath; cook for 50 minutes. Remove artichokes from the water bath and pat them dry. Then, blow torch artichokes to get the char marks.
4. Place artichokes on a serving platter.
5. In a bowl, mix the sour cream and mayonnaise. Serve artichokes with sour cream-mayo dip on the side. Bon appétit!

Nutrition Info: 314 Calories; 21g Fat; 21g Carbs; 3g Protein; 9g Sugars

Turkey In Orange Sauce

Servings: 2
Cooking Time: 42 Minutes;
Ingredients:
- 1 pound turkey breasts, skinless and boneless
- 1 tablespoon butter
- 3 tablespoons fresh orange juice
- ½ cup chicken stock
- 1 teaspoon Cayenne pepper, ground
- ½ teaspoon salt
- ¼ teaspoon black pepper, ground
- Serve with:
- Grilled eggplants

Directions:
1. Rinse the turkey breasts under cold running water and pat dry. Set aside.
2. In a medium bowl, combine orange juice, chicken stock, Cayenne pepper, salt, and pepper. Mix well and place the meat into this marinade. Refrigerate for 20 minutes.
3. Now, place the meat along with marinade into a large Ziploc bag and cook en sous vide for 40 minutes at 122 degrees.
4. In a medium nonstick saucepan, melt the butter over a medium-high temperature. Remove the meat from the bag and add it to the saucepan. Fry for about 2 minutes and remove from the heat.

Nutrition Info: Calories: 303 Total Fat: 9g Saturated Fat: 5g; Trans Fat: 0g Protein: 32g; Net Carbs: 13g

Salmon With Curried Tomatoes

Servings: 4
Cooking Time: 40 Minutes;
Ingredients:
- 2 pounds salmon fillets
- 1 cup grape tomatoes, diced
- 1 tablespoon red curry paste
- 3 tablespoons fresh basil, chopped
- tablespoons olive oil
- ½ teaspoon sea salt
- ¼ teaspoon black pepper, ground
- Serve with:
- Steamed asparagus

Directions:
1. Wash the grape tomatoes and finely dice. Set aside.
2. Rinse the salmon fillets under cold running water and pat dry with a kitchen paper. Gently rub the fillets with salt and pepper and place in a large Ziploc bag along with olive oil, basil, curry, and diced tomatoes. Seal the bag and cook en sous vide for 40 minutes at 131 degrees.

Nutrition Info: Calories: 444 Total Fat: 22g Saturated Fat: 4g; Trans Fat: 0g Protein: 45g; Net Carbs: 2g

Tasty French Toast

Servings: 2
Cooking Time: 100 Minutes
Ingredients:
- 2 eggs
- 4 bread slices
- ½ cup milk
- ½ tsp cinnamon
- 1 tbsp butter, melted

Directions:
1.   Prepare a water bath and place the Sous Vide in it. Set to 150 F.
2.   Whisk together the eggs, milk, butter and cinnamon. Place the bread slices in a vacuum-sealable bag and pour the egg mixture over. Shake to coat well. Release air by the water displacement method, seal and submerge the bag in water bath.Set the timer for 1 hour and 25 minutes. Once the timer has stopped, remove the bag. Serve warm.

Chicken Wings With Ginger

Servings: 4
Cooking Time: 2 Hours 25 Minutes
Ingredients:
- 2 pounds chicken wings
- ¼ cup extra virgin olive oil
- 4 garlic cloves
- 1 tbsp rosemary leaves, finely chopped
- 1 tsp white pepper
- 1 tsp cayenne pepper
- 1 tbsp fresh thyme, finely chopped
- 1 tbsp fresh ginger, grated
- ¼ cup lime juice
- ½ cup apple cider vinegar

Directions:
1.   Rinse the chicken wings under cold running water and drain in a large colander.
2.   In a large bowl, combine olive oil with garlic, rosemary, white pepper, cayenne pepper, thyme, ginger, lime juice, and apple cider vinegar. Submerge wings in this mixture and cover. Refrigerate for one hour.
3.   Transfer the wings along with the marinade in a large vacuum-sealable bag. Seal the bag and cook in sous vide for 1 hour and 15 minutes at 149 F.

Remove from the vacuum-sealable bag and brown before serving. Serve and enjoy!

Sweet And Sticky Tebasaki

Servings: 6
Cooking Time: 4 Hours 10 Minutes
Ingredients:
- 1 ½ pounds chicken drumettes
- Coarse sea salt and freshly ground black pepper, to your liking
- 3 tablespoons packed dark brown sugar
- 1 teaspoon ginger juice
- 1 tablespoon sake
- 1 tablespoon Shoyu sauce
- 1 teaspoon granulated garlic
- 1 tablespoon black vinegar
- 2 teaspoons sesame oil
- 2 tablespoons sesame seeds, toasted

Directions:
1.   Preheat a sous vide water bath to 148 degrees F.
2.   Now, season chicken drumettes with salt and black pepper.
3.   Place the seasoned chicken drumettes in cooking pouches; seal tightly.
4.   Submerge the cooking pouches in the water bath; cook for 4 hours.
5.   In a saucepan, heat the sugar, ginger juice, sake, Shoyu sauce, and granulated garlic over medium-high heat.
6.   Bring the sauce to a rolling boil; add the vinegar and allow this glaze to cool.
7.   Remove the chicken drumettes from the water bath; pat dry with kitchen towels.
8.   Heat the oil in a cast-iron skillet over medium-high heat; sear the chicken drumettes until well browned on both sides.
9.   Transfer the chicken drumettes directly to the bowl of glaze and toss to coat them completely. Serve garnished with toasted sesame seeds. Bon appétit!
Nutrition Info: 345 Calories; 26g Fat; 1g Carbs; 22g Protein; 3g Sugars

Winter Lamb Stew

Servings: 3

Cooking Time: 1 Hour
Ingredients:
- 1 pound lamb neck fillets
- 1 cup green beans, chopped
- 1 small red bell pepper, chopped
- 1 garlic clove, crushed
- 2 tablespoons extra-virgin olive oil
- 1 small carrot, chopped
- ¼ cup of lemon juice, freshly juiced
- ½ teaspoon salt
- ¼ teaspoon black pepper, ground
- Serve with:
- Cabbage salad

Directions:
1. Wash the meat under cold running water and pat dry with a kitchen paper. Cut into bite-sized pieces and rub with salt, pepper, garlic. Drizzle with lemon juice and set aside.
2. Wash the green beans and carrot. Cut into small pieces and set aside. Wash the bell pepper and cut in half. Remove the seeds and chop into small pieces. Set aside.
3. Place the meat along with vegetables and olive oil in a large Ziploc bag. Seal the bag and cook en sous vide for 1 hour at 154 degrees.

Nutrition Info: Calories: 399 Total Fat: 27g Saturated Fat: 5g; Trans Fat: 0g Protein: 49g; Net Carbs: 8g

Stuffed Collard Greens

Servings: 3
Cooking Time: 65 Minutes
Ingredients:
- 1 pound collard greens, steamed
- 1 pound lean ground beef
- 1 small onion, finely chopped
- 1 tbsp olive oil
- Salt and black pepper to taste
- 1 tsp fresh mint, finely chopped

Directions:
1. Boil a large pot of water and add in greens. Briefly cook, for 2-3 minutes. Drain and gently squeeze the greens and set aside.
2. In a large bowl, combine ground beef, onion, oil, salt, pepper, and mint. Stir well until incorporated.

Place leaves on your work surface, vein side up. Use one tablespoon of the meat mixture and place it in the bottom center of each leaf. Fold the sides over and roll up tightly. Tuck in the sides and gently transfer to a large vacuum-sealable bag. Seal the bag and cook in sous vide for 45 minutes at 167 F.

Italian-style Tomato Dipping Sauce

Servings: 10
Cooking Time: 45 Minutes
Ingredients:
- 2 pounds very ripe tomatoes, chopped with juices
- 1 cup scallions, chopped
- 3 cloves roasted garlic, pressed
- 2 teaspoons dried Italian herb seasoning
- 2 heaping tablespoons fresh cilantro, roughly chopped
- Sea salt and ground black pepper, to taste
- 1 teaspoon red pepper flakes
- 1 teaspoon sugar
- 2 tablespoons extra-virgin olive oil
- 1 cup Parmigiano-Reggiano cheese, preferably freshly grated

Directions:
1. Preheat a sous vide water bath to 180 degrees F.
2. Add all ingredients, minus cheese, to cooking pouches; seal tightly.
3. Submerge the cooking pouches in the water bath; cook for 40 minutes.
4. Place the prepared sous vide sauce in a serving bowl; top with grated Parmigiano-Reggiano cheese and serve with breadsticks. Bon appétit!

Nutrition Info: 71 Calories; 3g Fat; 6g Carbs; 3g Protein; 4g Sugars

Parmesan Chicken

Servings: 4
Cooking Time: 1 Hour
Ingredients:
- 1 pound chicken breast
- 1 tablespoon olive oil
- 1 small onion, finely chopped
- 2 garlic cloves, crushed

- 1 medium-sized red bell pepper, seeds removed and chopped
- ½ cup cauliflower, trimmed and chopped
- 1 teaspoon salt
- ½ teaspoon black pepper, ground
- 2 teaspoon fresh thyme, finely chopped
- 2 tablespoons tomato paste
- 1 tablespoon butter
- ½ cup Parmesan cheese
- Serve with:
- Fresh lettuce salad

Directions:

1. Wash and prepare the vegetables. Preheat the oil in a large skillet and sauté onions until translucent. Add chopped cauliflower and red bell pepper. Cook for about 3-4 minutes, or until vegetables are slightly tender. Add the butter and cook until melts, stirring constantly. Remove from the heat.

2. Now, wash the meat under cold running water and pat dry the meat with a kitchen paper. Chop the meat into bite-sized pieces and place in a large Ziploc bag along with vegetable mixture and all other ingredients. Seal the bag and cook en sous vide for 45 minutes at 167 degrees. Remove from the water bath and set aside to cool for a while before serving.

Nutrition Info: Calories: 352 Total Fat: 18g Saturated Fat: 6g; Trans Fat: 0g Protein: 39; Net Carbs: 5g

Traditional French Béarnaise Sauce

Servings: 12
Cooking Time: 45 Minutes
Ingredients:

- 4 tablespoons Champagne vinegar
- 1/2 cup dry white wine
- 1 tablespoon fresh tarragon, finely chopped
- 3 tablespoons shallots, finely chopped
- 5 egg yolks
- 2 sticks butter, melted
- 1 tablespoon fresh lemon juice

Directions:

1. Preheat a sous vide water bath to 148 degrees F.
2. In a pan, place the vinegar, wine, tarragon, and shallots; bring to a rolling boil.

3. Turn down heat to simmer. Continue cooking for 12 minutes.
4. Strain the mixture through a fine-mesh strainer into a food processor. Fold in the egg yolks and blitz mixture until uniform and smooth.
5. Place the sauce in cooking pouches; seal tightly. Submerge the cooking pouches in the water bath; cook for 25 minutes.
6. Add the contents from the cooking pouches to a mixing dish; add the butter and lemon juice; mix with an immersion blender until smooth.
7. Serve with your favorite roasted vegetable bites. Bon appétit!

Nutrition Info: 175 Calories; 12g Fat; 1g Carbs; 4g Protein; 3g Sugars

Vanilla Apricots With Whiskey

Servings: 4
Cooking Time: 45 Minutes
Ingredients:

- 2 apricots, pitted and quartered
- ½ cup rye whiskey
- ½ cup ultrafine sugar
- 1 tsp vanilla extract
- Salt to taste

Directions:

1. Prepare a water bath and place Sous Vide in it. Set to 182 F. Place all ingredients in a vacuum-sealable bag. Release air by the water displacement method, seal and submerge in water bath. Cook for 30 minutes. Once the timer has stopped, remove the bag and transfer into an ice bath.

Scallops With Bacon

Servings: 6
Cooking Time: 50 Minutes
Ingredients:

- 10 ounces scallops
- 3 ounces bacon, sliced
- ½ onion, grated
- ½ tsp white pepper
- 1 tbsp olive oil

Directions:

1. Prepare a water bath and place the Sous Vide in it. Set to 140 F.
2. Top the scallops with the grated onion and wrap with bacon slices. Sprinkle with white pepper and drizzle with oil. Place in a plastic bag. Release air by the water displacement method, seal and submerge the bag in water bath.Set the timer for 35 minutes. Once the timer has stopped, remove the bag. Serve.

Orange Duck With Paprika & Thyme

Servings: 4
Cooking Time: 15 Hours 10 Minutes
Ingredients:
- 16 ounces duck legs
- 1 tsp orange zest
- 2 tbsp Kaffir leaves
- 1 tsp salt
- 1 tsp sugar
- 1 tbsp orange juice
- 2 tsp sesame oil
- ½ tsp paprika
- ½ tsp thyme

Directions:
1. Prepare a water bath and place the Sous Vide in it. Set to 160 F. Dump all the ingredients in a vacuum-sealable bag. Massage to combine well. Release air by the water displacement method, seal and submerge the bag in water bath.Set the timer for 15 hours.
2. Once the timer has stopped, remove the bag. Serve warm.

Chicken Thighs With Green Beans

Servings: 3
Cooking Time: 1 Hour
Ingredients:
- 1 pound chicken thighs, boneless
- 1 cup green beans, chopped
- 2 garlic cloves, minced
- 1 teaspoon ginger, ground
- 1 tablespoon Cayenne pepper, ground
- 1 tablespoon lemon juice, freshly squeezed
- tablespoon olive oil
- ½ teaspoon salt
- 1 teaspoon fresh mint, finely chopped

- Serve with:
- Fresh tomatoes
Directions:
1. Wash the chicken thighs under cold running water and cut into thin slices. Gently rub the meat with salt, Cayenne pepper, and ginger. Set aside.
2. Wash the beans and chop into bite-sized pieces. Set aside.
3. Place the thighs along with beans, garlic, lemon juice, olive oil, and fresh mint in a large Ziploc bag. Seal the bag and cook en sous vide for 1 hour at 167 degrees.
4. Remove the bag from the water bath and set aside to cool for a while before serving.
Nutrition Info: Calories: 471 Total Fat: 33gSaturated Fat: 9g; Trans Fat: 0g Protein: 49g; Net Carbs: 9g

Chili Hummus

Servings: 9
Cooking Time: 4 Hours 15 Minutes
Ingredients:
- 16 ounces chickpeas, soaked overnight and drained
- 2 garlic cloves, minced
- 1 tsp sriracha
- ¼ tsp chili powder
- ½ tsp chili flakes
- ½ cup olive oil
- 1 tbsp salt
- 6 cups water

Directions:
1. Prepare a water bath and place the Sous Vide in it. Set to 195 F. Place the chickpeas and water in a plastic bag. Release air by the water displacement method, seal and submerge the bag in water bath.Set the timer for 4 hours.
2. Once the timer has stopped, remove the bag, drain the water and transfer the chickpeas to a food processor. Add in the remaining ingredients. Blend until smooth.

Easy Spiced Hummus

Servings: 6
Cooking Time: 3 Hours 35 Minutes

Ingredients:

- 1½ cups dried chickpeas, soaked overnight
- 2 quarts water
- ¼ cup lemon juice
- ¼ cup tahini paste
- 2 garlic cloves, minced
- 2 tbsp olive oil
- ½ tsp caraway seeds
- ½ tsp salt
- 1 tsp cayenne pepper

Directions:

1. Prepare a water bath and place the Sous Vide in it. Set to 196 F.
2. Strain the chickpeas and place in a vacuum-sealable bag with 1 quart of water. Release air by the water displacement method, seal and submerge the bag in the water bath. Cook for 3 hours. Once the timer has stopped, remove the bag and transfer into an ice water bath and allow to chill.
3. In a blender, mix the lemon juice and tahini paste for 90 seconds. Add in garlic, olive oil, caraway seeds, and salt, mix for 30 seconds until smooth. Remove the chickpeas and drain it. For a smoother hummus, peel the chickpeas.
4. In a food processor, combine the half of chickpeas with the tahini mix and blend for 90 seconds. Add the remaining chickpeas and blend until smooth. Put the mixture in a plate and garnish with cayenne pepper and the reserved chickpeas.

Braised Greens With Mint

Servings: 2
Cooking Time: 15 Minutes;
Ingredients:

- ½ cup fresh chicory, torn
- ½ cup wild asparagus, finely chopped
- ½ cup Swiss chard, torn
- ¼ cup fresh mint, chopped
- ¼ cup arugula, torn
- garlic cloves, minced
- ½ teaspoon salt
- tablespoons lemon juice, freshly squeezed
- 2 tablespoons olive oil
- Serve with:
- Sour cream

Directions:

1. Fill a large pot with salted water and add greens. Bring it to a boil and cook for 2-3 minutes. Remove from the heat and drain in a large colander. Gently squeeze with your hands and using a sharp knife chop the greens.
2. Transfer to a large Ziploc and cook en sous vide for 10 minutes at 162 degrees.
3. Remove from the water bath and set aside. Heat up the olive oil over medium-high heat in a large skillet. Add garlic and stir-fry for one minute. Now add greens and season with salt. Give it a good stir and remove from the heat.
4. Sprinkle with fresh lemon juice and serve warm or even cold.

Nutrition Info: Calories: 191 Total Fat: 11g Saturated Fat: 4g; Trans Fat: 0g Protein: 8g; Net Carbs: 4g

Beef Steak With Shallots And Parsley

Servings: 4
Cooking Time: 1 Hour
Ingredients:

- 1 large beef steak, about 2 pounds
- 2 tablespoons Dijon mustard
- 3 tablespoons olive oil
- 1 tablespoon fresh parsley leaves, finely chopped
- 1 teaspoon fresh rosemary, finely chopped
- 1 tablespoon shallot, finely chopped
- ½ teaspoon dried thyme
- 1 garlic clove, crushed
- Serve with:
- Red cabbage salad

Directions:

1. Clean the beef steak and cut into 1-inch thick slices. Set aside.
2. In a small bowl, combine Dijon mustard with olive oil. Add parsley, rosemary, shallot, thyme, and garlic. Rub the meat with this mixture and place in a Ziploc.
3. Cook en sous vide for one hour at 136 degrees for medium, or at 154 for well done.
4. Serve with red cabbage salad.

Nutrition Info: Calories: 521 Total Fat: 25g Saturated Fat: 9g; Trans Fat: 0g Protein: 63g; Net Carbs: 4g

Spicy Butter Corn

Servings: 5
Cooking Time: 35 Minutes
Ingredients:
- 5 tbsp butter
- 5 ears yellow corn, husked
- 1 tablespoon fresh parsley
- ½ tsp Cayenne pepper
- Salt to taste

Directions:
1. Prepare a water bath and place the Sous Vide in it. Set to 186 F.
2. Place 3 ears of corn in each vacuum-sealable bag. Release air by the water displacement method, seal and submerge the bags in the water bath. Cook for 30 minutes. Once the timer has stopped, remove the corn from the bags and transfer into a plate. Garnish with cayenne pepper and parsley.

Perfect Lil Smokies

Servings: 8
Cooking Time: 2 Hours
Ingredients:
- 2 pounds cocktail sausages
- 1 /12-ounce bottle chili sauce

Directions:
1. Preheat a sous vide water bath to 140 degrees F.
2. Add cocktail sausages and chili sauce to cooking pouches; seal tightly.
3. Submerge the cooking pouches in the water bath; cook for 2 hours.
4. Serve with toothpicks and enjoy!
Nutrition Info: 314 Calories; 24g Fat; 18g Carbs; 26g Protein; 5g Sugars

Dijon Chicken Filets

Servings: 4
Cooking Time: 65 Minutes
Ingredients:
- 1 pound chicken filets
- 3 tbsp Dijon mustard
- 2 onions, grated
- 2 tbsp cornstarch
- ½ cup milk
- 1 tbsp lemon zest
- 1 tsp thyme
- 1 tsp oregano
- Garlic salt and black pepper to taste
- 1 tbsp olive oil

Directions:
1. Prepare a water bath and place the Sous Vide in it. Set to 146 F. Whisk together all the ingredients and place in a vacuum-sealable bag. Release air by the water displacement method, seal and submerge the bag in water bath.Set the timer for 45 minutes. Once the timer has stopped, remove the bag and transfer to a saucepan and cook over medium heat for 10 minutes.

Classic Ragout

Servings: 3
Cooking Time: 1 Hour 20 Minutes;
Ingredients:
- 1 pound lamb chops, cut into 1-inch thick pieces
- 2 small carrots, finely chopped
- 1 medium-sized tomato, chopped
- ½ cup of green peas
- tablespoons extra-virgin olive oil
- ½ teaspoon salt
- ½ tablespoon Cayenne pepper, ground
- ¼ teaspoon black pepper, ground
- Serve with:
- Fresh lettuce salad

Directions:
1. Wash the lamb chops under cold running water and pat dry with a kitchen paper. Rub the lamb chops with salt, Cayenne pepper, and black pepper. Set aside.
2. Wash the carrots and tomato. Peel and chop into small pieces. Set aside.
3. Place the meat along with olive oil and green peas in a large Ziploc bag. Seal the bag and cook for 1 hour at 158 degrees.

4. Remove the bag from the water bath and set aside to cool for a while. Transfer all to a heavy-bottomed pot and add carrots and tomato. Add one cup of water and bring it to a boil. Reduce the heat to low and cover with a lid. Cook for 20 minutes and remove from the heat.

Nutrition Info: Calories: 492 Total Fat: 24g Saturated Fat: 6g; Trans Fat: 0g Protein: 46g; Net Carbs: 19g

Buttery & Sweet Duck

Servings: 7
Cooking Time: 7 Hours 10 Minutes
Ingredients:
- 2 pounds duck wings
- 2 tbsp sugar
- 3 tbsp butter
- 1 tbsp maple syrup
- 1 tsp black pepper
- 1 tsp salt
- 1 tbsp tomato paste

Directions:
1. Prepare a water bath and place the Sous Vide in it. Set to 175 F.
2. Whisk together the ingredients in a bowl and brush the wings with the mixture. Place the wings in a vacuum-sealable bag and pour over the remaining mixture. Release air by the water displacement method, seal and submerge the bag in water bath.Set the timer for 7 hours. Once the timer has stopped, remove the bag and slice. Serve warm.

Baby Carrots With Creamy Sesame Dressing

Servings: 6
Cooking Time: 1 Hour
Ingredients:
- 1 ½ pounds baby carrots
- Sea salt and white pepper, to taste
- 2 teaspoons olive oil
- 1 tablespoon fresh parsley, minced
- 1 tablespoon mint, minced
- Dressing:
- 1/3 cup sour cream

- 1 tablespoon lemon juice
- 1 teaspoon maple syrup
- 1/3 cup sesame seeds, toasted
- 1 tablespoon fresh dill leaves, chopped
- 1/2 teaspoon mustard powder

Directions:
1. Preheat a sous vide water bath to 183 degrees F.
2. Add baby carrots, salt, white pepper, olive oil, parsley, and mint to cooking pouches; seal tightly.
3. Submerge the cooking pouches in the water bath; cook for 55 minutes.
4. Now, make the dressing by mixing all ingredients.
5. Dress sous vide baby carrots and serve at room temperature. Enjoy!

Nutrition Info: 129 Calories; 1g Fat; 18g Carbs; 1g Protein; 6g Sugars

Lobster Tails

Servings: 6
Cooking Time: 50 Minutes
Ingredients:
- 1 pound lobster tails, pelled
- ½ lemon
- ½ tsp garlic powder
- ¼ tsp onion powder
- 1 tbsp rosemary
- 1 tsp olive oil

Directions:
1. Prepare a water bath and place the Sous Vide in it. Set to 140 F.
2. Season lobster with garlic and onion powder. Place in a vacuum-sealable bag. Add the rest of the ingredients and shake to coat. Release air by the water displacement method, seal and submerge the bag in water bath.Set the timer for 40 minutes. Once the timer has stopped, remove the bag. Serve warm.

Italian Chicken Fingers

Servings: 3
Cooking Time: 2 Hours 20 Minutes
Ingredients:
- 1 pound chicken breast, boneless and skinless
- 1 cup almond flour

- 1 tsp minced garlic
- 1 tsp salt
- ½ tsp cayenne pepper
- 2 tsps mixed Italian herbs
- ¼ tsp black pepper
- 2 eggs, beaten
- ¼ cup olive oil

Directions:

1. Rinse the meat under cold running water and pat dry with a kitchen paper. Season with mixed Italian herbs and place in a large vacuum-sealable. Seal the bag and cook in sous vide for 2 hours at 167 F. Remove from the water bath and set aside.

2. Now combine together flour, salt, cayenne, Italian herbs, and pepper in a bowl and set aside. In a separate bowl, beat the eggs and set aside.

3. Heat up olive oil in a large skillet, over medium heat. Dip the chicken into the beaten egg and coat with the flour mixture. Fry for 5 minutes on each side, or until golden brown.

Bacon-wrapped Turkey Leg

Servings: 5
Cooking Time: 6 Hours 15 Minutes
Ingredients:

- 14 ounces turkey leg
- 5 ounces bacon, sliced
- ½ tsp chili flakes
- 2 tsp olive oil
- 1 tbsp sour cream
- ½ tsp oregano
- ½ tsp paprika
- ¼ lemon, sliced

Directions:

1. Prepare a water bath and place the Sous Vide in it. Set to 160 F.

2. Combine in a bowl the herbs and spices with the sour cream and brush over the turkey. Wrap in bacon and drizzle with olive oil. Place in a vacuum-sealable bag along with lemon. Release air by the water displacement method, seal and submerge the bag in water bath. Set timer for 6 hours. Once the timer has stopped, remove the bag and slice. Serve warm.

Fresh Rosemary Chicken Thighs With Mushrooms

Servings: 4
Cooking Time: 40 Minutes;
Ingredients:

- 1 pound chicken thighs
- 1 cup button mushrooms, sliced
- tablespoons olive oil
- 1 teaspoon fresh rosemary, finely chopped
- 2 garlic cloves, crushed
- ½ teaspoon salt
- 1 tablespoon butter
- 1 tablespoon Italian seasoning mix
- Serve with:
- Fresh arugula

Directions:

1. Rinse well the meat under cold running water and rub with salt. Place in a large Ziploc bag along with olive oil, fresh rosemary, and salt. Cook en sous vide for 2 hours at 149 degrees.

2. Remove from the water bath and set aside.

3. Melt the butter in a large skillet, over medium-high heat. Add garlic and stir-fry for 2 minutes. Now add mushrooms and continue to cook for five more minutes. Finally, stir in Italian seasoning mix and remove from the heat.

4. Place chicken thighs on a serving plate and top with mushrooms.

Nutrition Info: Calories: 338 Total Fat: 29g Saturated Fat: 7g; Trans Fat: 0g Protein: 35g; Net Carbs: 3g

Radish Cheese Dip

Servings: 4
Cooking Time: 1 Hour 15 Minutes
Ingredients:

- 30 small radishes, green leaves removed
- 1 tbsp Chardonnay vinegar
- Sugar to taste
- 1 cup water for steaming
- 1 tbsp grapeseed oil
- 12 oz cream cheese

Directions:

1. Make a water bath, place Sous Vide in it, and set to 183 F. Put the radishes, salt, pepper, water, sugar, and vinegar in a vacuum-sealable bag. Release air from the bag, seal and submerge in the water bath. Cook for 1 hour. Once the timer has stopped, remove the bag, unseal and transfer the radishes with a little of the steaming water into a blender. Add cream cheese and puree to get a smooth paste. Serve.

Cod Bite Balls

Servings: 5
Cooking Time: 105 Minutes
Ingredients:
- 12 ounces minced cod
- 2 ounces bread
- 1 tbsp butter
- ¼ cup flour
- 1 tbsp semolina
- 2 tbsp water
- 1 tbsp minced garlic
- Salt and black pepper to taste
- ¼ tsp paprika

Directions:
1. Prepare a water bath and place the Sous Vide in it. Set to 125 F.
2. Combine the bread and water and mash the mixture. Add in the remaining ingredients and mix well to combine. Make balls out of the mixture.
3. Spray a skillet with cooking spray and cook the bite balls over medium heat about 15 seconds per side, until lightly toasted. Place the cod bites in a vacuum-sealable bag. Release air by the water displacement method, seal and submerge the bag in water bath. Set the timer for 1 hour and 30 minutes. Once the timer has stopped, remove the bag and plate the cod bites. Serve.

Green Pea Dip

Servings: 8
Cooking Time: 45 Minutes
Ingredients:
- 2 cups green peas
- 3 tbsp heavy cream
- 1 tbsp tarragon

- 1 garlic clove
- 1 tsp olive oil
- Salt and black pepper to taste
- ¼ cup diced apple

Directions:
1. Prepare a water bath and place the Sous Vide in it. Set to 185 F. Place all the ingredients in a vacuum-sealable bag. Release air by the water displacement method, seal and submerge the bag in water bath. Set the timer for 32 minutes. Once the timer has stopped, remove the bag and blend with a hand blender until smooth.

Asparagus With Garlic Dipping Sauce

Servings: 8
Cooking Time: 40 Minutes
Ingredients:
- 1 ½ pounds asparagus spears, halved lengthwise
- 1/2 stick butter, melted
- Sea salt and black pepper, to taste
- 4 garlic cloves, minced
- 1/2 cup plain yogurt
- 1/4 cup sour cream
- 1/4 cup mayonnaise
- 10 garlic cloves, smashed
- Salt and pepper, to taste

Directions:
1. Preheat a sous vide water bath to 183 degrees F.
2. Place asparagus spears, butter, salt, black pepper, and 4 garlic cloves in a large-sized cooking pouch; seal tightly.
3. Submerge the cooking pouch in the water bath; cook for 30 minutes.
4. In a bowl, mix the remaining ingredients to prepare a dipping sauce. Serve asparagus with garlic dipping sauce and enjoy!

Nutrition Info: 232 Calories; 15g Fat; 9g Carbs; 2g Protein; 7g Sugars

Herrings With Kale

Servings: 3
Cooking Time: 45 Minutes;
Ingredients:

- 1 pound herrings, cleaned
- 4 tablespoons extra virgin olive oil
- 2 tablespoons lime juice, freshly squeezed
- 1 teaspoon sea salt
- ¼ teaspoon red pepper flakes
- 1 tablespoon fresh basil, finely chopped
- 1 teaspoon dried thyme, ground
- 2 garlic cloves, crushed
- ¾ cup fresh kale
- 1 teaspoon butter
- Serve with:
- Greek yogurt

Directions:

1. Wash the fish under cold running water and place in a large bowl. Add oil, lime juice, salt, pepper, basil, thyme, and garlic. Rub each fish with this mixture and refrigerate for one hour.
2. Transfer to a large Ziploc bag along with the marinade and cook en sous vide for 40 minutes at 122 degrees.
3. Meanwhile, melt the butter in a medium-sized saucepan over a medium-high heat. Add kale and cook for five minutes, until tender. Remove from the heat and serve with fish.

Nutrition Info: Calories: 487 Total Fat: 38g Saturated Fat: 7g; Trans Fat: 0g Protein: 49g; Net Carbs: 3g

Oven Baked Yam Chips

Servings: 4
Cooking Time: 1 Hour 30 Minutes
Ingredients:

- 1 pound yams, peeled and cubed
- Coarse sea salt and freshly ground black pepper, to taste
- 2 tablespoons extra-virgin olive oil
- 1/2 teaspoon Hungarian paprika
- 1/3 teaspoon ancho chili powder

Directions:

1. Preheat a sous vide water bath to 183 degrees F.
2. Season the yams with salt and pepper.
3. Add the yams to a cooking pouch; seal tightly.
4. Submerge the cooking pouch in the water bath; cook for 60 minutes. Remove the yams from the cooking pouch and pat them dry.

5. Preheat an oven to 350 degrees F. Arrange the yams on a parchment-lined baking sheet in a single layer.
6. Drizzle olive oil over sous vide yams; sprinkle Hungarian paprika and ancho chili powder over them.
7. Bake approximately 25 minutes. Bon appétit!

Nutrition Info: 193 Calories; 9g Fat; 36g Carbs; 8g Protein; 6g Sugars

Ahi Tuna Steak

Servings: 4
Cooking Time: 45 Minutes;
Ingredients:

- 2 pounds Ahi tuna steaks
- ¼ cup fresh coriander, finely chopped
- 3 garlic cloves, minced
- 2 tablespoons lemon juice, freshly juiced
- 4 tablespoons olive oil
- ½ teaspoon smoked paprika
- ½ teaspoon cumin, ground
- ½ teaspoon salt
- ¼ teaspoon black pepper, ground
- Serve with:
- Steamed bell peppers

Directions:

1. Rinse the steaks under cold running water and pat dry with a kitchen paper. Set aside.
2. In a large bowl, combine olive oil, lemon juice, garlic, paprika, cumin, salt, and pepper. Mix well and add the meat. Coat the steaks and refrigerate for 30 minutes in this marinade.
3. Now, place all in a large Ziploc bag. Seal the bag and cook en sous vide for 45 minutes at 131 degrees. Remove the steaks from the bag and sprinkle with fresh coriander.

Nutrition Info: Calories: 545 Total Fat: 24g Saturated Fat: 7g; Trans Fat: 0g Protein: 62g; Net Carbs: 3g

Milky Mashed Potatoes With Rosemary

Servings: 4
Cooking Time: 1 Hour 45 Minutes
Ingredients:

- 2 pounds red potatoes
- 5 garlic cloves
- 8 oz butter
- 1 cup whole milk
- 3 sprigs rosemary
- Salt and white pepper to taste

Directions:

1. Prepare a water bath and place the Sous Vide in it. Set to 193 F. Wash the potatoes and peel them and slice. Take the garlic, peel and mash them. Combine the potatoes, garlic, butter, 2tbsp of salt, and rosemary. Place in a vacuum-sealable bag. Release air by the water displacement method, seal and submerge the bag in the water bath. Cook for 1 hour and 30 minutes.

2. Once the timer has stopped, remove the bag and transfer into a bowl and mash them. Stir the blended butter and milk. Season with salt and pepper. Top with rosemary and serve.

Shrimp Appetizer

Servings: 8
Cooking Time: 75 Minutes
Ingredients:

- 1 pound shrimps
- 3 tbsp sesame oil
- 3 tbsp lemon juice
- ½ cup parsley
- Salt and white pepper to taste

Directions:

1. Prepare a water bath and place the Sous Vide in it. Set to 140 F.

2. Place all ingredients in a vacuum-sealable bag. Shake to coat the shrimp well. Release air by the water displacement method, seal and submerge the bag in water bath.Set the timer for 1 hour. Once the timer has stopped, remove the bag. Serve warm.

Spicy Cauliflower Steaks

Servings: 5
Cooking Time: 35 Minutes
Ingredients:

- 1 pound cauliflower, sliced
- 1 tbsp turmeric

- 1 tsp chili powder
- ½ tsp garlic powder
- 1 tsp sriracha
- 1 tbsp chipotle
- 1 tbsp heavy
- 2 tbsp butter

Directions:

1. Prepare a water bath and place the Sous Vide in it. Set to 185 F.

2. Whisk together all of the ingredients, except cauliflower. Brush the cauliflower steaks with the mixture. Place them in a vacumm-sealable bag. Release air by the water displacement method, seal and submerge the bag in water bath.Set the timer for 18 minutes.

3. Once the timer has stopped, remove the bag and preheat your grill and cook the steaks for a minute per side.

Sweet Thighs With Sun-dried Tomatoes

Servings: 7
Cooking Time: 75 Minutes
Ingredients:

- 2 pounds chicken thighs
- 3 ounces sun dried tomatoes, chopped
- 1 yellow onions, chopped
- 1 tsp rosemary
- 1 tbsp sugar
- 2 tbsp olive oil
- 1 egg, beaten

Directions:

1. Prepare a water bath and place the Sous Vide in it. Set to 149 F.

2. Combine all the ingredients in a vacuum-sealable bag and shake to coat well. Release air by the water displacement method, seal and submerge the bag in water bath.Set the timer for 63 minutes. Once the timer has stopped, remove the bag and serve as desired.

Creamy And Cheesy Seafood Dip

Servings: 12
Cooking Time: 40 Minutes
Ingredients:

- 6 ounces scallops, chopped
- 6 ounces shrimp, chopped
- 2 cups broth, preferably homemade
- 1 ½ cups Colby cheese, shredded
- 1 ½ cups Gruyere cheese, shredded
- 1/2 teaspoon smoked paprika
- 1/2 teaspoons ground black pepper
- 1/2 teaspoon dried oregano

Directions:

1. Preheat a sous vide water bath to 132 degrees F.
2. Simply put all ingredients into cooking pouches; seal tightly.
3. Submerge the cooking pouches in the water bath; cook for 35 minutes.
4. Transfer the sous vide dipping sauce to a nice serving bowl; serve with dippers of choice. Bon appétit!

Nutrition Info: 206 Calories; 12g Fat; 2g Carbs; 25g Protein; 2g Sugars

Mini Pork Carnitas

Servings: 12
Cooking Time: 18 Hours 10 Minutes
Ingredients:

- 3 pounds boneless pork butt
- Sea salt and ground black pepper, to taste
- 2 garlic cloves, smashed
- 1 habanero pepper, deseeded and minced
- 1 cup ale
- 1/2 cup bone broth
- 1 teaspoon dried basil
- 1 teaspoon dried rosemary
- 2 bay leaves
- 24 wonton wraps
- 1 cup Queso Manchego, shredded
- 1 cup Pico de gallo, for garnish

Directions:

1. Preheat a sous vide water bath to 145 degrees F.
2. Place pork, salt, pepper, garlic, habanero pepper, ale, bone broth, basil, rosemary, and bay leaves in cooking pouches; seal tightly.
3. Submerge the cooking pouches in the water bath; cook for 18 hours. Remove sous vide pork from the cooking pouches and shred with two forks.

4. Preheat your oven to 380 degrees F. Spritz a mini muffin pan with a nonstick cooking spray.
5. Fill wonton wraps with shredded pork. Top with shredded Queso Manchego. Bake about 9 minutes.
6. Remove from the oven; allow them to cool for 5 minutes before serving. Serve with Pico de gallo on the side. Bon appétit!

Nutrition Info: 405 Calories; 24g Fat; 14g Carbs; 34g Protein; 5g Sugars

Jarred Pumpkin Bread

Servings: 4
Cooking Time: 3 Hours 40 Minutes
Ingredients:

- 1 egg, beaten
- 6 tbsp canned pumpkin puree
- 6 ounces flour
- 1 tsp baking powder
- 1 tsp cinnamon
- ¼ tsp nutmeg
- 1 tbsp sugar
- ¼ tsp salt

Directions:

1. Prepare a water bath and place the Sous Vide in it. Set to 195 F.
2. Sift the flour along with the baking powder, salt, cinnamon, and nutmeg in a bowl. Stir in beaten egg, sugar and pumpkin puree. Mix to form a dough.
3. Divide the dough between two mason jars and seal. Place in water bath and cook for 3 hours and 30 minutes. Once the time passed, remove the jars and let it cool before serving.

Party-friendly Mini Sliders

Servings: 8
Cooking Time: 3 Hours 15 Minutes
Ingredients:

- 1/2 pound ground pork
- 1/2 pound ground sirloin
- Sea salt and freshly ground black pepper, to taste
- 1 /25-ounce envelope onion soup mix
- 4 tablespoons mayonnaise
- 1 tablespoon Dijon mustard

- 1 banana shallot, chopped
- 3/4 pound Gorgonzola cheese, crumbled
- 16 miniature burger buns

Directions:

1. Preheat a sous vide water bath to 145 degrees F.
2. Thoroughly combine ground meat, salt, pepper, and envelope onion soup mix in a mixing dish.
3. Shape the mixture into 16 meatballs with your hands. Flatten each portion into a small patty, about 1/2-inches-thick.
4. Transfer the prepared patties to cooking pouches; seal tightly.
5. Submerge the cooking pouches in the water bath; cook for 3 hours.
6. Heat a grill pan over medium-high flame. Grill burgers for 1 to 2 minutes on each side, working in batches.
7. Divide the mayonnaise, mustard and shallot among the bottom buns. Now, top each with a slider, and finish with Gorgonzola cheese. Cover with the top of the bun and serve immediately.

Nutrition Info: 314 Calories; 24g Fat; 18g Carbs; 26g Protein; 5g Sugars

DESSERTS RECIPES

Lemon Curd

Servings: 8
Cooking Time: 75 Minutes
Ingredients:
- 1 cup butter
- 1 cup sugar
- 12 egg yolks
- 5 lemons

Directions:
1. Prepare a water bath and place the Sous Vide in it. Set to 168 F.
2. Grate the zest from lemons and place in a bowl. Squeeze the juice and add to the bowl as well. Whisk on the yolks and sugar and transfer to a vacumm-sealable bag. Release air by the water displacement method, seal and submerge the bag in water bath.Set the timer for 1 hour.
3. Once the timer has stopped, remove the bag and transfer the cooked lemon curd to a bowl and place in an ice bath. Let chill completely.

Mesmerizing Chia Pudding Pots

Servings: 2
Cooking Time: 60 Minutes
Ingredients:
- 120g of chia seeds
- 4 cups of coconut milk
- 2 tablespoon of honey
- 4 drops of vanilla extract
- 1 cup of mango puree
- 2 tablespoon of sliced coconut flesh

Directions:
1. Carefully prepare your sous vide water bath to a temperature of 140° Fahrenheit using the immersion cooker
2. Take a heavy duty re-sealable bag and add chia seeds, honey, coconut milk and vanilla
3. Seal it up using immersion method and place it under your pre-heated water and cook for about 75 minutes
4. Remove your bag from the water and divide it amongst 4 bowls

5. Top up each of your dish with coconut mango and sprinkle some chia seeds
6. Serve!
Nutrition Info: Calories: 145 Fat 4g, Protein 4g, Dietary Fiber 5g

Vanilla & Butter Pears

Servings: 2
Cooking Time: 30 Minutes
Ingredients:
- 2 peeled ripe pears
- 1 vanilla bean
- 2 tablespoons dark brown sugar
- 1/8 teaspoon flaky sea salt
- 1 tablespoon unsalted butter
- Vanilla ice cream for serving

Directions:
1. Set up your Sous Vide immersion circulator to a temperature of 175-degrees Fahrenheit and prepare your water bath.
2. Slice the pears in half lengthwise.
3. Scoop out the core using a spoon, divide the pear halves between two resealable bags.
4. Then, cut/slice the vanilla bean in half and use the back of the spoon to scrape its seeds into a small bowl.
5. Add the brown sugar and salt.
6. Then, rub the vanilla bean seed into sugar using your fingers and combine.
7. Divide the mixture between the resealable bags and add 1 tablespoon of butter and one half of your vanilla pod into each bag.
8. Seal using the immersion method. Cook for 30 minutes.
9. Remove the bag from the water bath. Take the pears out from the bag and then transfer to serving bowls.
10. Drizzle the butter sauce from the bag over the pears and serve with vanilla ice cream.
Nutrition Info: Per serving:Calories: 441 ;Carbohydrate: 109g ;Protein: 1g ;Fat: 1g ;Sugar: 90g ;Sodium: 10mg

Chili Agave Liqueur

Servings: 8
Cooking Time: 45 Minutes
Ingredients:
- 2 cups vodka
- ½ cup water
- ½ cup light agave nectar
- 3 dried Guajillo chili peppers
- 1-piece Serrano pepper, sliced in half and seeded
- 1 Fresno pepper, sliced in half and seeded
- Zest of 1 lemon
- 1 cinnamon stick
- 1 teaspoon black peppercorns

Directions:
1. Prepare your Sous Vide water bath using your immersion circulator and raise the temperature to 180-degrees Fahrenheit.
2. Add all the listed ingredients to a heavy-duty zip bag.
3. Seal using the immersion method and cook for 45 minutes.
4. Once done, remove the bag and strain the contents to a bowl.
5. Transfer to liquid storage, chill and serve!
Nutrition Info: Calories: 139 Carbohydrate: 37g Protein: 1g Fat: 0g Sugar: 29g Sodium: 8mg

Cinnamon Apples

Cooking Time: 40 Mins Cooking Temperature: 185°f
Ingredients:
- 4 medium apples, peeled, cored and sliced
- 1 tablespoon brown sugar
- 2 tablespoons unsalted butter
- ¼ teaspoon ground cinnamon

Directions:
1. Attach the sous vide immersion circulator using an adjustable clamp to a Cambro container or pot filled with water and preheat to 185°F.
2. Into a bowl, add all ingredients and toss to coat well.
3. Into a cooking pouch, add apple slices in a single layer. Seal pouch tightly after squeezing out the excess air. Place pouch in sous vide bath and set the cooking time for 30-40 minutes.

4. Remove pouch from sous vide bath and carefully open it. Transfer apple mixture onto a plate and serve immediately.

Butter & Sea Salt Radish

Servings: 4
Cooking Time: 45 Minutes
Ingredients:
- 1 lb. halved radishes
- 3 tablespoons unsalted butter
- 1 teaspoon sea salt
- ½ teaspoon freshly ground black pepper

Directions:
1. Prepare your Sous Vide water bath using your immersion circulator and raise the temperature to 180-degrees Fahrenheit.
2. Take a medium-sized resealable bag and add all the listed ingredients to the bag
3. Seal it using the immersion method and let it cook underwater for about 45 minutes.
4. Once cooked, remove the bag and transfer the contents to a platter.
5. Serve!
Nutrition Info: Per serving:Calories: 302 ;Carbohydrate: 43g ;Protein: 9g ;Fat: 12g ;Sugar: 4g ;Sodium: 352mg

Bacon Vodka

Servings: 10
Cooking Time: 45 Minutes
Ingredients:
- 2 cups vodka
- 8 oz. bacon
- 3 tablespoons reserved bacon grease

Directions:
1. Prepare your Sous Vide water bath using your immersion circulator and raise the temperature to 150-degrees Fahrenheit.
2. Bake the bacon for 16 minutes at 400-degrees Fahrenheit.
3. Allow the mixture to cool.
4. Add all the ingredients to a resealable bag and seal using the immersion method.
5. Cook for 45 minutes.

6. Strain the liquid into bowl and chill until a fat layer forms.
7. Remove and skim off the fat layer, strain using a cheesecloth once again.
8. Serve chilled!

Nutrition Info: Calories: 295 Carbohydrate: 9g Protein: 5g Fat: 17g Sugar: 4g Sodium: 572mg

Rice Pudding With Rum & Cranberries

Servings: 6
Cooking Time: 2 Hours 15 Minutes
Ingredients:
- 2 cups rice
- 3 cups milk
- ½ cup dried cranberries soaked in ½ cup of rum overnight and drained
- 1 tsp cinnamon
- ½ cup brown sugar

Directions:
1. Prepare a water bath and place the Sous Vide in it. Set to 140 F.
2. Combine all the ingredients in a bowl and transfer to 6 small jars. Seal them and submerge in water bath.Set the timer for 2 hours. Once the timer has stopped, remove the jars. Serve warm or chilled.

Citrus Yogurt

Servings: 4
Cooking Time: 180 Minutes
Ingredients:
- ½ cup yogurt
- ½ tablespoon orange zest
- ½ tablespoon lemon zest
- ½ tablespoon lime zest
- 4 cups full cream milk

Directions:
1. Set up your Sous Vide immersion circulator to a temperature of 113-degrees Fahrenheit and prepare your water bath.
2. Heat the milk on stove top to a temperature of 180-degrees Fahrenheit.
3. Transfer to an ice bath and allow it to cool down to 110-degrees Fahrenheit.
4. Stir in yogurt.

5. Fold in the citrus zest.
6. Pour the mixture into 4-ounce canning jars and lightly close the lid.
7. Submerge underwater and cook for 3 hours.
8. Remove the jars and serve immediately!

Nutrition Info: Per serving:Calories: 175 ;Carbohydrate: 35g ;Protein: 6g ;Fat: 2g ;Sugar: 32g ;Sodium: 66mg

Mint Julep & Coconut Sugar

Servings: 2
Cooking Time: 90 Minutes
Ingredients:
- 2 cups water
- 2 cups bourbon
- 1 ½ cups coconut sugar
- 2 cups fresh mint

Directions:
1. Prepare your Sous Vide water bath using your immersion circulator and raise the temperature to 135-degrees Fahrenheit.
2. Add the water, coconut sugar, bourbon, and mint to a resealable zip bag.
3. Seal using the immersion method.
4. Cook for 1 ½ hour.
5. Strain and serve chilled!

Nutrition Info: Calories: 124 Carbohydrate: 5g Protein: 0g Fat: 0g Sugar: 4g Sodium: 0mg

Flourless Chocolate Cake

Servings: 6
Cooking Time: 60 Minutes
Ingredients:
- 1/2 cup unsalted butter
- 4 ounces bittersweet chocolate
- 3/4 cup sugar
- 3 large eggs /lightly beaten
- 2 tablespoons coffee liqueur
- 1/2 cup unsweetened cocoa powder
- Powdered sugar /for garnish

Directions:
1. Preheat water to 115°F in a sous vide cooker or with an immersion circulator.

2. For the batter, in a microwave or double boiler, melt chocolate and butter, stirring until smooth. Whisk sugar into batter mixture until smooth. Add eggs and liqueur and whisk until combined. Sift cocoa powder over batter and whisk until combined.

3. Spray six 4-ounce canning jars with nonstick cooking spray. Pour batter into jars and screw on lids fingertip-tight. Submerge jars in water and cook for 1 hour.

4. Remove jars from water, let cool on a wire rack to room temperature and refrigerate until chilled through, at least 6 hours. Cakes can be stored in the refrigerator, covered, for up to 10 days.

5. About 30 minutes before serving, turn cakes out of jars onto dessert plates /use a thin knife to loosen cakes from jars if necessary. Sift powdered sugar over cakes and serve. Enjoy!

Nutrition Info: Calories: 386; Total Fat: 25g; Saturated Fat: 15g; Protein: 6g; Carbs: 40g; Fiber: 5g; Sugar: 33g

Rum Bananas

Servings: 4
Cooking Time: 30 Minutes
Ingredients:
- 4 large bananas, sliced
- 1 cup brown sugar
- 1 tablespoon pineapple juice
- 1 tablespoon dark rum

Directions:
1. Heat the Sous Vide cooker to 175F.
2. Combine the bananas, sugar, pineapple juice, and rum into a Sous Vide bag.
3. Vacuum seal the bag and submerge in water.
4. Cook 30 minutes.
5. Finishing steps:
6. Remove the bag from the cooker.
7. Open carefully and transfer into dessert bowls.
8. Serve at room temperature.

Nutrition Info: Calories 269 Total Fat 5g Total Carb 61g Dietary Fiber 6g Protein 5g

Spiced Coconut Ice Cream

Servings: 4

Cooking Time: 30 Minutes
Ingredients:
- 1 can (13 oz.) full-fat coconut milk
- ¾ cup sugar
- ½ teaspoon kosher salt
- 2 teaspoons vanilla extract
- ½ teaspoon ground cinnamon
- ¼ teaspoon nutmeg
- ¼ teaspoon coriander
- 4 large egg yolks
- Tools required
- Ice Cream Maker

Directions:
1. Set up your Sous Vide immersion circulator to a temperature of 180-degrees Fahrenheit and prepare your water bath.
2. Take a medium-sized saucepan and add the coconut milk, salt, sugar, cinnamon, vanilla, nutmeg, coriander and bring it to a simmer.
3. Once done, remove the heat and allow it to steep for 30 minutes.
4. Transfer to a blender and purée the mixture alongside the egg yolks for 30 seconds
5. Transfer the mixture to a resealable zip bag and seal using the immersion method.
6. Cook for 30 minutes, making sure to agitate the bag from time to time.
7. Chill the bag in an ice bath and churn the mixture in an ice cream maker.
8. Freeze and serve!

Nutrition Info: Per serving:Calories: 693 ;Carbohydrate: 36g ;Protein: 9g ;Fat: 60g ;Sugar: 32g ;Sodium: 183mg

Ginger Crème Brûlée

Cooking Time: 55 Mins Cooking Temperature: 185°f
Ingredients:
- ⅔ cup whole milk
- 2 cups heavy whipping cream
- 4 teaspoons peeled and fresh chopped ginger
- 4 large egg yolks
- ½ cup superfine sugar
- pinch of salt

Directions:

1. Attach the sous vide immersion circulator using an adjustable clamp to a Cambro container or pot filled with water and preheat to 185°F.
2. Into a medium pan add milk, cream and ginger, and warm through on a low heat.
3. Remove from heat and allow liquid to steep for 30 minutes.
4. Through a fine mesh sieve, strain the mixture and discard the solids.
5. Return the liquid to another pan and cook until just heated.
6. Into a bowl, add egg yolks and beat well.
7. Slowly add sugar and salt, beating continuously.
8. Slowly add ginger mixture, beating continuously until well-combined.
9. Place ⅔ cup of mixture into each ramekin. With a piece of plastic wrap, cover each ramekin and secure with a rubber band.
10. Carefully arrange ramekins over the rack in sous vide bath (water level should come ⅔ up the sides of the ramekins). Set the cooking time for 50 minutes.
11. Carefully, remove ramekins from sous vide bath onto wire rack to cool slightly.
12. Remove plastic wrap and keep aside to cool completely.
13. After cooling, refrigerate until chilled.
14. Before serving, spread a thin layer of sugar on top of each chilled custard. With a torch, caramelize top of each custard.
15. Serve immediately.

Blueberry Clafoutis

Servings: 4
Cooking Time: 60 Minutes
Ingredients:
- 1 piece of whole egg
- ¼ cup of heavy cream
- ¼ cup of almond flour
- 1 tablespoon of granulated sugar
- 2 teaspoon of coconut flour
- ¼ teaspoon of baking powder
- ¼ teaspoon of vanilla extract
- Just a pinch of salt
- ½ a cup of fresh blueberries

- 4 pieces of 4 ounce screw top – hinge closure canning jar
Directions:
1. Set your water bath to 185° Fahrenheit
2. Tale a small bowl and add all of the ingredients except blueberries
3. Set up your jars on your work surface and grease with some cooking spray
4. Divide the prepared batter evenly among the 4 jars
5. Top it up with 2 tablespoon of blueberries
6. Attach the lids with fingertip lightness /to ensure that the air is able to escape once submerged under water
7. Put them in your water bat and cook for 1 hour
8. Remove the jar from the bath and open it up
9. Enjoy warm with a sprinkle of sugar or crème anglaise
Nutrition Info: Calories: 228, Fat 3g, Protein 5g, Dietary Fiber 2g

Pumpkin Bread

Cooking Time: 3 Hours Cooking Temperature: 195°f
Ingredients:
- 1 cup all-purpose flour
- 1 teaspoon baking powder
- ¼ teaspoon baking soda
- 2 teaspoons ground cinnamon
- ½ teaspoon ground nutmeg
- pinch of ground cloves
- ½ cup vegetable oil
- ⅓ cup granulated sugar
- ¼ cup dark brown sugar
- ¾ cup canned pumpkin puree
- ½ teaspoon salt
- 2 large eggs
Directions:
1. Attach the sous vide immersion circulator using an adjustable clamp to a Cambro container or pot filled with water and preheat to 195°F.
2. Generously grease 4 half-pint canning jars.
3. In a bowl, mix together flour, baking powder, baking soda and spices.
4. In another bowl, add oil, both sugars, pumpkin puree and salt and beat until well-combined.

5. Add eggs, one at a time, beating until well-combined.

6. Add flour mixture into pumpkin mixture, and mix until just combined.

7. Divide mixture evenly into prepared jars. (Each jar should be not full more than two-thirds full).

8. With a damp towel, wipe off sides and tops of jars. Tap the jars onto a counter firmly to remove air bubbles.

9. Close each jar. (Do not over-tighten jars because air will need to escape).

10. Place jars in sous vide bath and set the cooking time for 3 hours.

11. Remove the jars from sous vide bath and carefully remove the lids. Place jars onto a wire rack to cool completely.

12. Carefully run a knife around the inside edges of the jars to loosen the bread from the walls.

13. Cut into slices and serve.

Almond Nectarine Pie

Servings: 6
Cooking Time: 3 Hours 20 Minutes
Ingredients:

- 3 cups nectarines, peeled and diced
- 8 tbsp butter
- 1 cup sugar
- 1 tsp vanilla extract
- 1 tsp almond extract
- 1 cup milk
- 1 cup flour

Directions:

1. Prepare a water bath and place the Sous Vide in it. Set to 194 F. Grease small jars with cooking spray. Gather the nectarines amongst the jars.

2. In a bowl, mix sugar and butter. Add the almond extract, whole milk and vanilla extract, mix well. Stir the self-rising flour and blend until solid. Place the batter into the jars. Seal and submerge the jars in the water bath. Cook for 180 minutes. Once the timer has stopped, remove the jars. Serve.

Cherry Cheesecake

Cooking Time: 1 Hour 35 Mins Cooking Temperature: 176°f
Ingredients:

- For Topping:
- 2 cups fresh cherries, pitted
- ¼ cup granulated sugar
- cornstarch, as required
- whipped cream, as required
- For Cheesecake:
- Graham cracker crumbs, as required
- 16 ounces Philadelphia cream cheese
- ½ cup granulated sugar
- ¼ cup heavy cream
- 1 tablespoon vanilla extract
- 2 eggs, lightly beaten

Directions:

1. For the topping:

2. add cherries to a pan over a medium heat and cook until they begin to release their liquid. Stir in sugar and bring to a boil, stirring occasionally.

3. Reduce heat and simmer until cherries become tender.

4. Slowly add cornstarch, stirring continuously.

5. Cook until mixture becomes thick, stirring continuously.

6. Remove from heat and keep aside to cool.

7. Attach the sous vide immersion circulator using an adjustable clamp to a Cambro container or pot filled with water and preheat to 176°F.

8. For the cheesecake:

9. arrange a thin layer of Graham cracker crumbs into the bottom of your desired number of canning jars.

10. Into the bowl of an electric mixer, place cream cheese and beat until slightly softened.

11. Add sugar, heavy cream and vanilla extract, and beat until well-combined.

12. Add half of the beaten eggs, and beat until well-combined.

13. Add the remaining beaten eggs, and beat until well-combined and smooth.

14. Place the cream cheese mixture evenly into the jars.

15. Screw the canning jar lids closed tightly. Carefully arrange jars into sous vide bath and set the cooking time for 1½ hours.
16. Carefully, remove jars from sous vide bath and place onto a wire rack to cool slightly.
17. After cooling, refrigerate to chill completely.
18. Remove the lid from each jar and place cherry topping evenly over each cheesecake.
19. Top with whipped cream and serve.

Minty Vodka Melon

Servings: 4
Cooking Time: 2 Hours 10 Minutes
Ingredients:
- 1 cup melon chunks
- 1 cup vodka
- 12 mint leaves
- 1 tsp sugar

Directions:
1. Prepare a water bath and place the Sous Vide in it. Set to 140 F. Place all the ingredients in a jar and mix to combine. Seal and submerge the jar in water bath. Set the timer for 2 hours. Once the timer has stopped, remove the jar. Strain and serve.

Tomato Shrub

Servings: 12
Cooking Time: 1 Hour 30 Minutes
Ingredients:
- 2 cups diced tomatoes
- 2 cups granulated sugar
- 2 cups red wine vinegar
- 1 cup water

Directions:
1. Prepare your Sous Vide water bath using your immersion circulator and raise the temperature to 180-degrees Fahrenheit.
2. Add all the listed ingredients to a resealable zip bag and seal using the immersion method.
3. Cook for 1 ½ hour.
4. Once done, remove and strain the contents into a bowl.
5. Discard any solids and transfer to storing jar.
6. Serve as needed!

Nutrition Info: Calories: 126 Carbohydrate: 30g Protein: 1g Fat: 0g Sugar: 28g Sodium: 80mg

Sous Vide Chocolate Cupcakes

Servings: 6
Cooking Time: 3 Hours 15 Minutes
Ingredients:
- 5 tbsp butter, melted
- 1 egg
- 3 tbsp cocoa powder
- 1 cup flour
- 4 tbsp sugar
- ½ cup heavy cream
- 1 tsp baking soda
- 1 tsp vanilla extract
- 1 tsp apple cider vinegar
- Pinch of sea salt

Directions:
1. Prepare a water bath and place the Sous Vide in it. Set to 194 F. Whisk together the wet ingredients in one bowl. Combine the dry ingredients in another bowl. Combine the two mixtures gently and divide the batter between 6 small jars. Seal the jars and submerge the bag in water bath. Set the timer for 3 hours Once the timer has stopped, remove the bag. Serve chilled.

Incredible Coffee Dessert

Servings: 8
Cooking Time: 3 Hours 10 Minutes
Ingredients:
- 1/3 cup espresso
- ¾ cup milk
- 1 cup heavy cream
- 6 oz white chopped chocolate
- 1/3 cup sugar
- ½ tsp salt
- Whipped cream
- 4 large egg yolks

Directions:
1. Prepare a water bath and place the Sous Vide in it. Set to 182 F.

2.   Heat a saucepan over medium heat and stir the heavy cream, espresso and milk. Remove from the heat and add the chocolate. Cook for 15 minutes.

3.   Combine egg yolks, salt, and sugar in a bowl. Mix in the chocolate mixture. Allow cooling. Place the mixture in a vacuum-sealable bag. Release air by water displacement method, seal and submerge in the bath. Cook for 30 minutes. Once done, transfer contents to small ramekins. Chill for 2 hours.

Vanilla Cheesecake

Servings: 6
Cooking Time: 1 Hour 45 Minutes
Ingredients:
- 12 oz cream cheese, at room temperature
- ½ cup sugar
- ¼ cup mascarpone, at room temperature
- 2 eggs
- Zest of 1 lemon
- ½ tbsp vanilla extract

Directions:
1.   Prepare a water bath and place the Sous Vide in it. Set to 175 F.

2.   Combine cream cheese, mascarpone and sugar. Mix well. Stir in the eggs. Add in lemon zest and vanilla extract. Mix well. Pour the mixture in 6 mason jars. Seal and submerge in the water bath. Cook for 90 minutes. Once the timer has stopped, remove the jars and allow chilling. Top with fruit compote.

Orange Cheesy Mousse

Servings: 8
Cooking Time: 1 Hour 25 Minutes
Ingredients:
- 2 cups milk
- 6 tbsp white wine vinegar
- 4 oz chocolate chips
- ¼ cup powdered sugar
- Grand Marnier liquor
- 1 tbsp orange zest
- 2 oz goat cheese

Directions:
1.   Prepare a water bath and place the Sous Vide in it. Set to 172 F.

2.   Place the milk and vinegar in a vacuum-sealable bag. Release air by the water displacement method, seal and submerge the bag in the water bath. Cook for 60 minutes.

3.   Once the timer has stopped, remove the bag and reserve the curds. Discard the remaining liquid. Strain the curds for 10 minutes. Allow chilling for 1 hour.

4.   Prepare a water bath to medium heat and add the chocolate chips. Cook until melted. Transfer to a blender and stir the sugar, orange zest, grand Marnier, goat cheese. Mix until smooth. Serve into individual bowls.

Mulled Wine

Servings: 2
Cooking Time: 60 Minutes
Ingredients:
- ½ bottle red wine
- Juice of 2 oranges, peel of 1
- 1 cinnamon stick
- 1 bay leaf
- 1 vanilla pod, sliced in half lengthways
- 1-star anise
- 2 oz. caster sugar

Directions:
1.   Prepare your Sous Vide water bath using your immersion circulator and raise the temperature to 140-degrees Fahrenheit.

2.   Add all the listed ingredients to a large bowl.

3.   Divide the mixture across two resealable zip bags and seal using the immersion method. Cook for 1 hour.

4.   Serve chilled!

Nutrition Info: Calories: 206 Carbohydrate: 17g Protein: 1g Fat: 0g Sugar: 11g Sodium: 0mg

Banana Buckwheat Porridge

Servings: 4
Cooking Time: 12 Hours 15 Minutes
Ingredients:
- 2 cups buckwheat
- 1 banana, mashed
- ½ cup condensed milk

- 1 tbsp butter
- 1 tsp vanilla extract
- 1 ½ cup water
- ¼ tsp salt

Directions:

1. Prepare a water bath and place the Sous Vide in it. Set to 180 F.
2. Place the buckwheat in a vacumm-sealable bag. Whisk the remaining ingredients in a bowl. Pour this mixture over the buckwheat. Release air by the water displacement method, seal and submerge the bag in water bath.Set the timer for 12 hours.
3. Once the timer has stopped, remove the bag. Serve warm.

Dulce De Leche Cheesecake

Servings: 6
Cooking Time: 5 Hours 55 Minutes + 4 Hours
Ingredients:

- 2 cups mascarpone, at room temperature
- 3 eggs
- 1 tsp almond extract
- 1 cup dulce de leche
- ⅓ cup heavy cream
- 1 cup graham cracker crumbs
- 3 tbsp butter, melted
- ½ tsp salt

Directions:

1. Prepare a water bath and place the Sous Vide in it. Set to 175 F.
2. With an electric mixer, mix the mascarpone, eggs, and almond in a bowl until smooth. Pour 3/4 cup of dulce de leche and mix well. Add in cream and stir until fully combined. Set aside.
3. Combine the graham cracker crumbs and melted butter. Divide the crumbs mixture into six mini mason jars. Pour cream cheese mixture over the crumbs. Seal with a lid and submerge the jars in the water bath, Cook for 1 hour and 30 minutes.
4. Once the timer has stopped, remove the jars and transfer into the fridge and allow to cool for 4 hours. Top with the remaining dulce de leche. Garnish with the salted caramel mixture.

Honey Baked Cheese

Servings: 6
Cooking Time: 50 Minutes
Ingredients:

- 2 cups milk
- 6 tbsp white wine vinegar
- 2 large eggs
- 2 tbsp olive oil
- Salt and black pepper to taste
- 2 tbsp honey to serve

Directions:

1. Prepare a water bath and place the Sous Vide in it. Set to 172 F. Place the vinegar and milk in a vacuum-sealable bag. Release air by the water displacement method, seal and submerge the bag in the water bath. Cook for 60 minutes.
2. Preheat the oven to 350 F. Once the timer has stopped, remove the bag and strain the cuds. Allow to draining for 10 minutes. Transfer to a blender and mix with the eggs, salt, olive oil and pepper for 20 seconds. Put the ricotta in 6 oven ramekins and bake for 30 minutes. Sprinkle with honey.

Swedish Rosemary Snaps

Servings: 10
Cooking Time: 120 Minutes
Ingredients:

- 1 bottle vodka
- 3 sprigs fresh rosemary + plus extra for storage
- 4 strips of fresh orange peel

Directions:

1. Prepare your Sous Vide water bath using your immersion circulator and raise the temperature to 135-degrees Fahrenheit.
2. Add the vodka, 3 sprigs rosemary, and 3 strips of orange peel to a resealable zip bag.
3. Seal using the immersion method. Cook for 2 hours.
4. Once done, take the bag out from the water bath and pass through metal mesh strainer into large bowl.
5. Put one fresh sprig of rosemary and one strip of orange peel into bottle.
6. Pour the prepared snaps into bottle.
7. Chill and serve!

Nutrition Info: Calories: 236 Carbohydrate: 14g Protein: 0g Fat: 0g Sugar: 11g Sodium: 4mg

Nutrition Info: Calories: 256 Carbohydrate: 30g Protein: 4g Fat: 1g Sugar: 16g Sodium: 23mg

Vanilla Cava Fudge

Servings: 6
Cooking Time: 60 Minutes
Ingredients:
- 1 cup whipping cream
- ½ cup cava
- ½ cup sugar
- 4 egg yolks
- 1 tsp vanilla extract
- ½ tsp salt

Directions:
1. Prepare a water bath and place the Sous Vide in it. Set to 194 F. Blend all the ingredients for 30 seconds. Place it in a vacuum-sealable bag. Release air by the water displacement method, seal and submerge the bag in the water bath.
2. Cook for 45 minutes. Once the timer has stopped, remove the bag and transfer into an ice-water bath. Serve immediately.

Asian-style Rice Pudding With Almonds

Servings: 5
Cooking Time: 7 Hours 30 Minutes
Ingredients:
- 5 tbsp basmati rice
- 2 (14-oz) cans coconut milk
- 3 tbsp sugar
- 5 cardamom pods, crushed
- 3 tbsp cashews, chopped
- Slivered almonds for garnish

Directions:
1. Prepare a water bath and place the Sous Vide in it. Set to 182 F.
2. In a bowl, combine the coconut milk, sugar, and 1 cup water. Pour the rice and mix well. Divide the mixture between the jars. Add a cardamom pod to each pot. Seal and submerge in the bath. Cook for 3 hours. Once the timer has stopped, remove the jars. Allow cooling for 4 hours. Serve and top with cashews and almonds.

Strawberry & Rhubarb Shrub

Servings: 12
Cooking Time: 1 Hour 30 Minutes
Ingredients:
- 2 cups granulated sugar
- 2 cups balsamic vinegar
- 1 cup diced rhubarb
- 1 cup strawberries, diced
- 1 cup water

Directions:
1. Prepare your Sous Vide water bath using your immersion circulator and raise the temperature to 180-degrees Fahrenheit.
2. Add all the listed ingredients to a large-sized heavy-duty zip bag
3. Seal using the immersion method and cook for 1 ½ hour.
4. Remove the bag and strain the contents to a bowl.
5. Save the fruit for later.
6. Transfer to liquid storage, chill and serve!

Lemon Curd Pie

Servings: 8
Cooking Time: 45 Minutes
Ingredients:
- 1 prepared pie crust
- ¼ cup butter, melted
- Juice of 4 lemons
- 6 egg yolks
- 1 cup sugar
- Whipped cream for serving

Directions:
1. Preheat the water bath to 180°F.
2. Whisk together sugar, butter, and lemon juice, then whisk in egg yolks.
3. Pour mixture into a bag and seal. Place bag in the water bath and cook 45 minutes.
4. Pour curd into prepared pie crust. Cover with plastic wrap. Transfer to refrigerator and cool overnight.

5. Top chilled pie generously with whipped cream and serve.

Nutrition Info: Calories 246 Total Fat 128g Total Carb 267g Dietary Fiber 4g Protein 51g

Peach With Lavender

Cooking Time: 20 Mins Cooking Temperature: 185°f

Ingredients:

- 2 peaches, halved and pitted
- ¼ cup honey
- ¼ cup water
- 1 tablespoon dried lavender buds

Directions:

1. Attach the sous vide immersion circulator using an adjustable clamp to a Cambro container or pot filled with water and preheat to 185°F.
2. Into a cooking pouch, add all ingredients. Seal pouch tightly after squeezing out the excess air. Place pouch in sous vide bath and set the cooking time for 20 minutes.
3. Remove pouch from sous vide bath and immediately plunge into a large bowl of ice water for 15-20 minutes.
4. Open the pouch and transfer peaches into a bowl. Through a fine-mesh sieve, strain the poaching liquid into a bowl. Discard the lavender buds.
5. Serve chilled peach halves chilled, along with pouching liquid.

Wine And Cinnamon Poached Pears

Servings: 4

Cooking Time: 80 Minutes

Ingredients:

- 4 pears, peeled
- 2 cinnamon sticks
- 2 cups red wine
- 1/3 cup sugar
- 3 star anise

Directions:

1. Prepare a water bath and place the Sous Vide in it. Set to 175 F.

2. Combine the wine, anise, sugar, and cinnamon in a large vacumm-sealable bag. Place the pears inside. Release air by the water displacement method, seal and submerge the bag in water bath.Set the timer for 1 hour. Once the timer has stopped, remove the bag. Serve the pears drizzle with the wine sauce.

The Cobbler Of Peach

Servings: 6

Cooking Time: 180 Minutes

Ingredients:

- 3 cups of peeled and diced freestone peaches
- 8 tablespoon of unsalted butter
- 1 cup of granulated sugar
- 1 teaspoon of vanilla extract
- 1 teaspoon of almond extract
- 1 cup of whole milk
- 1 cup of self-rising flour

Directions:

1. Carefully prepare your sous vide water bath to a temperature of 195° Fahrenheit using the immersion cooker
2. Spray the inside of your 235ml canning jars with cooking spray
3. Divide the freestone peaches evenly amongst your jars
4. Take a medium sized bowl and use an electric mixer, add sugar and butter and mix them for about 5 minutes on medium settings
5. Lower down the mixer to low speed and add almond extract, vanilla extract, whole milk and mix everything well to combine them well
6. Add your self raising flour and combine well to make sure no lumps are formed
7. Pour the batter evenly amongst your jars
8. Seal up the lids loosely
9. Place the jars under your water bath and let them cook for about 180 minutes
10. 1 Remove the jars once done
11. 1 Open up the lid and brown the top just a bit by using a blowtorch
12. 1 Serve your cobblers hot!

Nutrition Info: Calories: 525 Fat: 19g, Protein: 6g, Dietary Fiber: 3g

APPENDIX : RECIPES INDEX

Crispy Skinned Salmon 72
Crunchy Apple Salad With Almonds 25
Curry Ginger & Nectarine Chutney 13
Curry Mackerel 77

D

Delicious Artichokes With Simple Dip 85
Delicious Cardamom And Apricots 13
Delicious Chicken Wings With Buffalo Sauce 50
Dijon & Curry Ketchup Beef Sausages 61
Dijon Chicken Filets 91
Divine Garlic-lemon Crab Rolls 77
Drunken Beef Steak 57
Dublin-style Lemon Shrimp Dish 73
Duck Leg Confit 35
Dulce De Leche Cheesecake 107

E

Easy Garden Green Beans 25
Easy Spiced Hummus 89
Easy Tilapia 81
Easy Vegetable Alfredo Dressing 15
Easy-to-make Tenderloin With Cayenne Sauce 61
Eggplant Lasagna 18

F

Fall Squash Cream Soup 10
Fire-roasted Tomato Tenderloin 61
Fish Tacos 75
Flavorful Pork With Mustard & Molasses Glaze 53
Flavorful Vegan Stew With Cannellini Beans 10
Flourless Chocolate Cake 101
Fresh Rosemary Chicken Thighs With Mushrooms 93
Fried Chicken 44

G

Garlic & Paprika Sweet Potatoes 28
Ginger Crème Brûlée 102
Ginger Tamari Brussels Sprouts With Sesame 14
Grape Vegetable Mix 6
Greek Meatballs With Yogurt Sauce 63
Green Beans & Mandarin Hazelnuts 23
Green Chicken Salad With Almonds 48
Green Pea Cream With Nutmeg 17
Green Pea Dip 94

H

Hearty White Beans 17

Herb Crusted Lamb Rack 63
Herby Balsamic Mushrooms With Garlic 7
Herby Braised Leeks 22
Herby Chicken With Butternut Squash Dish 43
Herby Lemon Salmon 82
Herrings With Kale 94
Honey Apple & Arugula Salad 9
Honey Baked Cheese 107
Honey Drizzled Carrots 8
Honey Flavored Chicken Wings 37
Honey Kumquats 27
Honey Mustard Pork 52
Honey Poached Pears 26

I

Incredible Coffee Dessert 105
Italian Chicken Fingers 92
Italian-style Fruit Toast 27
Italian-style Tomato Dipping Sauce 87

J

Jarred Pumpkin Bread 97
Jerk Pork Ribs 57

K

Kimchi Rib Eye Tacos With Avocado 60

L

Lamb Shank With Veggies & Sweet Sauce 62
Lazy Man's Lobster 77
Lemon Curd 99
Lemon Curd Pie 108
Lemony & Peppery Flank Steak 59
Lightly Seasoned Beets 19
Lobster Rolls 81
Lobster Tails 92
Loin Pork With Almonds 68
Lollipop Lamb Chops 68
Long Green Beans In Tomato Sauce 9

M

Ma Po Tofu 24
Mango Salsa & Pork 63
Maple Beet Salad With Cashews & Queso Fresco 16
Mashed Potato 31
Mesmerizing Chia Pudding Pots 99
Milky Mashed Potatoes With Rosemary 95
Mini Pork Carnitas 97
Mint Julep & Coconut Sugar 101
Minted Lamb Chops With Nuts 59
Minty Sardines 83

CPSIA information can be obtained
at www.ICGtesting.com
Printed in the USA
LVHW111609040222
710245LV00004B/51

9 781801 668521